Writing on the Job

Books of Related Interest

WRITING ON THE JOB

A Guide for Nurse Managers

KATHLEEN GARVER MASTRIAN, R.N., M.N.
Instructor in Nursing
The Pennsylvania State University
Shenango Valley Campus
Sharon, Pennsylvania

ERIC BIRDSALL, Ph.D.
Associate Professor of English
The Pennsylvania State University
Shenango Valley Campus
Sharon, Pennsylvania

A Wiley Medical Publication
JOHN WILEY & SONS
New York • Chichester • Brisbane • Toronto • Singapore

Library of Congress Cataloging-in-Publication Data:
Mastrian, Kathleen Garver.
  Writing on the job.

  (A Wiley medical publication)
  Includes index.
  1. Nursing service administration. 2. Nursing—
Authorship. I. Birdsall, Eric, 1944– .
II. Title. III. Series. [DNLM: 1. Administrative
Personnel. 2. Writing Personnel. WY 105 M423w]
RT89.M393 ' 1986   362.1'73'068   85-18005
ISBN 0-471-82174-8

Printed in the United States of America

10 9 8 7 6 5 4 3 2 1

To

Robert and Rosalie Garver
Angelo and Jennie Mastrian
Kathryn Birdsall
and the memory of
Reed Birdsall

Preface

Writing is an unnatural act. The process of translating our thoughts into words and getting those words onto paper can be one of the most difficult, threatening, and foreign of human tasks. Most people would rather do almost anything than write—take out the garbage, wash the car, scrub the floor, paint the house, take a walk, go to a movie: humans are endlessly inventive in finding things to do instead of write. That's because people aren't stupid. Writing is hard work, so they find ways to put it off.

Almost no one really *enjoys* writing, even people who do it a lot. "Well," you might say, "you people wrote a book so you must enjoy writing." Nope. We often like what happens after we've written: people sometimes learn from our work, enjoy it, or pay us for it. Those are all nice things. And once in a while, when we're lucky enough to locate just the right word or shape a really good sentence, we experience a little surge of satisfaction. But those rewards are rare. For us as for most people, writing remains a rugged, troublesome task, not something we choose for enjoyment.

For nurse managers, we've discovered, writing is even harder than for some other professionals. To see why, think back on the writing that was emphasized in your education and work as a staff nurse. In almost every case, you learned to do as little writing as possible, even to the extent of avoiding complete sentences. Good charting involves something akin to shorthand: recording information accurately but also as succinctly as possible. CCU, GI, TPR, PRN: all testify to the nurse's continuing quest to spend as little time as possible writing in order to leave as much time as possible for quality patient care. This special kind of writing is difficult and important. Doing it well requires a special skill. But it's highly adapted to a particular environment and not very useful in general communication.

By the time you reach a management position, therefore, you're accustomed to writing that is incomprehensible except to other health care professionals. One of the perversities of achieving a management position is that you have to write more and more as you assume increasingly responsible positions. And you no longer communicate with just physicians and other nurses. You eventually have to write to a wide variety of people, both inside your institution and outside: vendors, other administrators, patients and their families, lawyers, assorted bureaucrats, accrediting agency officials, and others. You've come a far distance from assessments, care plans, and charts.

WHAT THIS BOOK WILL DO (AND WON'T)

We've written this book to be a guide, a manual that you'll read through, then use as needed. We want to give you *advice*, not instructions. You'll find us emphasizing *content* over form and *process* over product. Therefore, you'll find very few prescriptions in our book (or, more precisely, *your* book). Effective writing results from clear thinking, thorough preparation, and good sense. Practice helps, too, along with some occasional direction. We'll show you many examples of good writing and some that are less good, and we'll explain why they're effective or not. We hope you'll think about both kinds of examples and how they might relate to your own writing.

HOW TO USE THIS BOOK

You may be tempted to turn directly to the chapter that discusses the kind of writing you do most (or have to do tomorrow). We hope you won't. The book is arranged from general to specific, from theory to practice. The more general chapters come first, and they provide the basis and much explanation for what follows. So please read them first. They'll help you understand an approach to writing that we're sure will help you every day.

Our approach is called *reader-centered writing*. We didn't invent it. Teachers of advanced composition and business and professional writing have been telling their college and university classes about it for a few years now. But we have not seen it applied specifically to the writing nursing managers are required to do. The process calls for you to pay attention to three elements in any writing situation: your *topic*, your *purpose*, and especially your *reader*. Most writers don't spend nearly enough time understanding the *people* to whom they'll be writing. But good writing is like good conversation. It requires a clear awareness of the other person.

We have tried to practice what we preach, so this book probably sounds different than most of the scholarly and professional writing you read. Imagining real readers holding the book, we have tried to make it interesting and accessible. You will find a lot of words (like *we* and *you*) and an informal style that you don't usually encounter in your professional reading. As we discuss in Chapter 3, good writing isn't inflated or stuffy. We could have written in a more impersonal style and said *It is suggested that the reader consider the following points* instead of *We suggest that you think about these things*. But big words and a distant style don't always aid effective communication. In fact, they often get in the way. We hope this book communicates person to person, us to you.

If you apply the reader-centered process of writing intelligently, you're likely to produce a good document. Because each writing task is different in large or small ways from every other, you should design each document specifically for the reader(s) and purpose(s) it's to serve. That's why we don't offer you lots of forms and "pattern" documents: what works well in one situation may fail in another.

In the last half of the book, you'll find discussions of some of the specific kinds of writing nurse managers do regularly. You'll find more examples there—generally good, we think—but remember that it's the *process* of writing that's important, not the form of any example we may show you. No doubt we'll sometimes say things with which you disagree, perhaps even that you know aren't true for you or your work setting. When that happens, please sift out what doesn't apply but hold onto what does. Throughout the book, of course, you should evaluate what we say. If it seems to make sense, try it. If it doesn't, don't. Experiment. Be creative. In short, use the book in any way that works for you.

KATHLEEN GARVER MASTRIAN
ERIC BIRDSALL

Acknowledgments

This book results from a true collaboration. Chapters 1–4 were drafted by Eric Birdsall and 6–9 by Kathleen Mastrian. We both read every word of every chapter; sometimes we read, argued, revised, and read again. Fittingly enough, our individual efforts merged at the center of the book in Chapter 5, which contains sections originally written separately then brought together, and in our samples for analysis in Chapter 10. But the entire book is a joint effort, and we must accept equal responsibility for its errors of commission, ommission, and judgment.

No one completes any book without incurring many debts, not all of them, alas, acknowledged or even remembered. We are aware of some of ours. Eric Birdsall completed his work while on sabbatical from The Pennsylvania State University, to which he is grateful for its support. Our editors at John Wiley—Andrea Stingelin, Janet Walsh Foltin, and Bruce Williams—have been unfailingly friendly, supportive, and helpful. All authors should be so lucky. Our students at Penn State contributed more than they probably realize; we often learned from them, and they forced us to redefine and clarify what we had to say. Laura DeBonis, Paula Reiber, and Marlene Hopkins typed parts of the manuscript quickly, accurately, and more cheerfully than we sometimes deserved. Chip, Trez, Benjamin, Alicia, and Kate haven't always known what we were doing, but they tolerated our foolishness with patience and grace.

Our most important obligations are recorded in the dedication. We regret that Reed Birdsall wasn't able to see the book. We think he would have gruffed a bit but liked it just the same.

KATHLEEN GARVER MASTRIAN
ERIC BIRDSALL

Sharon, Pennsylvania

Contents

Writing
on the Job

1

Consider Your Reader

In this chapter, we'll begin our discussion of the writing you do on the job with some background. We'll explain some basic communication theory. Then we'll ask you to think about how to bring together the three essential elements of writing an effective document: your reader, your topic, and your purpose. You'll find that you already know much of what we have to say because it's based largely on common sense, and you weren't promoted to management because you lack common sense or because you're a bad communicator. But if you're like most people, you may not know *that* you know *what* you know, and you probably haven't thought much about how these matters relate to the writing you have to do on the job.

THE COMMUNICATION PROCESS

The process of communication, people used to think, is quite simple. The writer determines what needs to be said, chooses the right words to convey her meaning, and sends them to her audience. In this view,

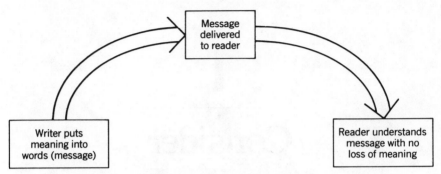

Figure 1.1.   A simplified model of the communication process.

the communicator's responsibility is simply to pack all his meaning into the message before it is delivered to the recipient, rather like someone packing a suitcase—if it's done carefully enough, the cargo will emerge intact and unwrinkled. The recipient then gets the message (unpacks the suitcase) and understands precisely what the communicator meant. Figure 1.1 depicts this concept of communication.

One problem with this concept is that it reduces the writer or speaker to a somewhat mechanical role: someone who packages a message into a neat container that is then delivered to the audience. The recipient opens the box, plucks out the tidy message, and understands everything perfectly. Communication, this model suggests, is as simple as saying what's on your mind, and it therefore emphasizes only one end of the process—the person who originates the message. The *meaning* seems to be the same as the *message*. Yet if you think a moment, you'll see that communication really isn't that simple at all. Unfortunately, an audience can, and often does, fail to understand even the most carefully crafted messages. Think about something as simple as a conversation in the hall between acquaintances. Even if we're discussing uncomplicated topics, we must constantly adjust for the possibility of misunderstanding with the person to whom we're speaking. He or she doesn't understand, so we restate a point. She or he asks a question; we answer. In the constant give-and-take of conversation, we constantly "read" and adapt to our audience, making many small adjustments when our messages are not understood clearly.

The problems of misunderstanding are much more difficult when we must address a group that can't give us verbal clues that our meaning is not being understood. And the most difficult situation of all occurs when we must write to an audience we can't see at all.

The simplified view of communication reflected in Figure 1.1 focuses upon the writer (or speaker) rather than the reader (or audience) and therefore leads most people into two common errors. First, they fail to take into account the actual, sometimes frustrating complexities of communication, especially writing. In real situations, we cannot usually transmit our meaning simply and directly in neat little boxes. Communication is untidy and difficult, and most messages cannot possibly transmit our actual meanings without misunderstanding. Effective communication involves much more than simply delivering a message. A second common error occurs when we blame the receiver for any misunderstanding. Such a response is common, for we almost always know what we mean, and a reader who fails to apprehend it must be too stupid, too busy, or too stubborn to understand what we have said. Yet communication of any kind is always a two-way transaction, and problems are not exclusively the reader's. In fact, it seems much more sensible to locate principal responsibility for ensuring effective communication on the originator of the message—the speaker or writer. As writers, we must undertake to solve the many problems of conveying our *meaning* (not just a message) to the audience. For it is we who know what we want to say, to whom we will be saying it, under what circumstances, and so on. In short, the person most responsible for effective communication must be you, the writer.

About 40 years ago, during the World War II, communications theorists began to develop a more sophisticated understanding of the communications process. Experts began to understand that the *message* is not the same thing as the *meaning* because many factors can interfere with the transfer of meaning from one person to another, preventing readers from understanding the meaning we intend to convey. Communications theory continues to develop rapidly, and we need not understand all its recent changes in order to put it to work for us as writers and speakers. One version of recent theory is illustrated in Figure 1.2. In this newer model, the originator of a message (the writer) has a meaning to be expressed but cannot communicate it directly to a reader. The writer must first "encode" the meaning into a message to be sent to the

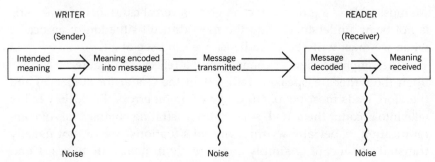

Figure 1.2. A more accurate model of the communication process, showing how noise can interfere.

reader. Such a message may take the form of Morse code sent by a te-legrapher, nurse's notes written in a patient's chart, or a detailed 15-page budget presentation with graphs and statistical tables. In every case, the writer must *encode* the intended meaning in order to send it, and the vehicle that carries the meaning is not the meaning itself. Some senders are better at encoding messages than others, but everyone can improve with practice.

Electronics engineers who studied communications for the military and space program quickly recognized the important problem of *noise,* or unwanted interference with the communications process. Sometimes this noise is precisely that—actual static that obscures a radio, television, or microwave message. But while a radio operator, for example, must worry about thunderstorms and other forms of external interference, the writer confronts a different problem. The kinds of "noise" that can in-terfere with written communication are many and distressingly varied: bad grammar, misspellings, poor organization, sloppy thinking—all of these can hinder communication. And this is just from the writer's end of the process.

When the message finally reaches the reader, he or she must *decode* the message back into a meaning. The reader, like a secret agent with a cryptogram, must interpret the message in order to understand its meaning. As with the writer, so too is the reader subject to confusing noise. If you as a reader are tired, confused by the subject, unfriendly toward the writer, or simply miss an important point, the communications process will break down even more, and even less of the message will be translated into meaning accurately. Sometimes, indeed, the distractions caused by noise can become so severe that the sender's meaning will become completely unintelligible, with the reader failing to understand, or—and this is sometimes worse—misunderstanding what the writer has intended. *Noise,* therefore, means any of the factors that can interfere with the efficient encoding and decoding of the message that passes from writer to reader.

As you can readily see, much can happen between the writer encoding a meaning into a message and the reader decoding the message at the end of the process. By now, it must seem that writers experience limitless ways to have messages go wrong and almost no chance of communicating anything clearly. But take heart. We need not become telegraphers or communications engineers in order to put this communications model to work for us as writers. The value of the model is that it demonstrates that no matter what you *mean,* and even no matter what message you *send,* all that matters is the decoded meaning that your reader finally *receives.* Effective writers, therefore, will not focus principally on themselves but on *readers.* It is your responsibility as a writer to do whatever you can to eliminate troublesome noise and to design a message that will convey your meaning as clearly as possible.

The principal problem with the communications model shown in Figure 1.2 is that it doesn't help us understand *how* readers actually decode the messages they receive. To know that would require a detailed understanding of cognitive psychology and thinking processes that most readers lack, certainly including the Nursing and English instructors who have written this book. But we can offer some observations about how readers respond to certain kinds of written messages and suggestions about how to guide readers to an understanding of the meaning you want them to receive. The three most important parts of the writing process we want you to be able to use are these:

- Clarify your goals.
- Understand your audience.
- Write reader-based prose that aims at a particular person or group of people.

CLARIFYING YOUR GOALS

Every message has a purpose—the reason it was written. (We assume that no sane person chooses to write merely to pass the time; there are many better ways to do that.) Before you write, decide what your purpose is—what goal do you hope to achieve by writing? It may be simply to inform someone, to entertain, to educate, to influence, to persuade. Or it may be some combination of these. Ask yourself these questions:

- Why am I writing this?
- What do I want my reader(s) to do when they read it?

Is your message intended to inform the nursing staff about a new procedure? If so, your purpose is to inform, and you want the reader to understand the new procedure. Do you want to change people's minds about something? Do you want to inform patients about how to take a medication and then persuade them to do it? Do you want to persuade the administration to purchase a new piece of equipment for your unit?

Often messages that we write at work will have multiple purposes, but until you have decided precisely *why* you are writing, you cannot hope to create an effective message. Consider the following example. Imagine you are a head nurse. In the course of your professional reading, you have come across an advertisement for a piece of equipment that you might consider recommending for purchase. However, you need further information, so you write a short letter to the manufacturer:

Widgetcorp., Inc.
2880 National Highway
Quahog, NY 14855

Gentlemen:

I recently saw an advertisement for the SuperWidget Mark II psychomotor regulator in *Head Nurse Magazine.*

Please send me information on performance specifications (including recycling time), cost, and any other material you think might be useful to me. Also, please include a list of nearby hospitals that are using the SuperWidget Mark II.

Yours truly,

Donna Wilson, R.N.
Head Nurse

Your purpose, of course, is merely to gain additional information about a piece of equipment that seems interesting, and your letter is admirably clear and straightforward. The following example shows the sort of reply such a letter might receive from many businesses.

Dear Ms. Wilson:

We are in receipt of your letter of November 28 concerning the SuperWidget Mark II.

Please be advised that the SuperWidget Mark II is in wide use in hospitals such as yours.

Enclosed please find our brochure which I am sure will answer your questions. The SuperWidget Mark II is available in both portable and permanent-installation configurations.

If I can be of further assistance, please do not hesitate to contact me.

Sincerely,

E. B. Sahl

This bland, thoughtless reply indicates that the writer took as his purpose only to answer an inquiry as effortlessly as possible. Sahl's letter is obviously an all-purpose form letter that reveals no attention or sensitivity to Wilson's request—or to the opportunity it offers Widgetcorp. Consider how much more effective a revised version would have been:

Dear Ms. Wilson:

Thank you for writing about the SuperWidget Mark II. As the enclosed information indicates, the SuperWidget is comparable in price to other psychomotor regulators but offers you much more.

Its recycling time is .05 seconds, considerably faster than the usual .20 seconds of similar equipment. This means faster turnaround time with patients and more effective use of valuable nurses' time.

In addition, the new technology in the SuperWidget makes it extremely accurate and reliable. We have recently installed units at Sagamon Valley Hospital and Lakeview Community Hospital. I hope you will contact your colleagues about their reaction to the SuperWidget.

Printed materials alone cannot reveal all the features of the SuperWidget, so I have asked Walter Johnson, our upstate New York representative, to contact you for an appointment. Mr. Johnson will be happy to demonstrate the SuperWidget to you and your staff.

Once you see the SuperWidget in operation, I am sure you will agree that it offers the best combination of features available today. Thank you for your interest in SuperWidget.

Sincerely,

E. B. Sahl

The revision addresses Wilson's questions directly, points out features of the machine that are likely to interest her, and takes an action that might very well lead to a sale (assuming that the SuperWidget is as good as Sahl claims). The letter is superior because Sahl has considered carefully his purpose in writing (to persuade as well as inform Wilson) and has tailored his message to the needs of a specific reader.

UNDERSTANDING YOUR AUDIENCE

A really effective piece of communication will always be written to a specific audience, be it one person or a large group. Only when you have a clear understanding of both your own purposes as a writer *and* the characteristics of your audience can you create a message that is likely to be understood fully and have the desired effect. Sometimes such obvious characteristics as age, sex, or personal background will be important because of interests and concerns that will be common to all or most people in a particular group. We might assume that most undertakers, for example, have shared interests that we might take into account in writing to one of them or a group of them. In most cases, however, the important features of an audience you must address will become clear only after careful analysis.

In general, you will need to consider three characteristics of your intended audience:

- What does your audience *know* about your topic?
- What are its *attitudes* toward your topic?
- What are its personal or professional *needs?*

In each case, the audience's knowledge, attitudes, and needs are likely to be different from yours. The careful writer will seek to understand the nature and degree of these differences in order to decrease the distance between reader and writer. Let's look more closely at these three areas.

Knowledge: What does your reader know about your topic? What does he or she need to know in order to understand or do what you want? What, if anything, do you hope to teach? In how much detail? Does the reader have the necessary background to understand you fully? If not, can you modify what you have to say? In short, does the reader have (or can you supply) enough information to achieve your goals?

Attitudes: How does your reader view your topic? Is he or she sympathetic? antagonistic? indifferent? How does the reader view you? What preconceptions or misinformation might your reader have? Is the reader skeptical? Willing to be persuaded? Already persuaded? What sort of approach is most likely to build upon favorable attitudes or reduce unfavorable feelings? Whether your purpose is to persuade or just to explain, you need to understand the beliefs and attitudes your reader holds. As an example, imagine that you have identified a new piece of equipment that will certainly improve the quality of care in your geriatric unit. It costs $2500, and you will need three. It will not make nursing care more cost-effective (that is, it won't enable the same number of nurses to take care of more patients), but it will help a significant number of patients both physically and psychologically. To see how differences in attitude can affect your writing, imagine how differently two individuals would respond to the suggestion that you purchase the three pieces of equipment: the head nurse on the unit and the head of the hospital's budget control committee. Clearly, the budget person will have attitudes that would make him or her much more difficult to convince than the head nurse. The more the reader's attitudes differ from your own, the more carefully you must craft your message.

Needs: When you consider the needs of the reader, you determine how to adapt what you have to say to him or her. While it is possible to change readers' attitudes, their needs are more or less fixed and should be acommodated. As an example, consider the differences between what a nurse records on a patient's chart and what she or he tells the patient. In one case, the needs of other nurses and physicians dictate that certain kinds of information be communicated in certain ways, while similar sorts of information (and perhaps even different information) will be communicated in different ways to the patient. As another example, read the messages concerning the drug Aldomet (methyldopa) below. The first is an information sheet for patients who will be taking the medication for the first time, the other a pharmacologic description from Loebl et al., *The Nurse's Drug Handbook*, 3d ed. (Wiley, 1983).

Patient Medication Information Sheet

MEDICATION TRADE NAME   Aldomet

USE   Treatment of hypertension (high blood pressure). Hypertension must be controlled in order to minimize the danger of long-term complications such as stroke, heart disease, and kidney disease.

DOSE

ADDITIONAL INSTRUCTIONS

    1. Take your medication as directed. Take it regularly and do not change the dosage, as this may reduce the drug's effectiveness.

    2. Have your blood pressure checked regularly, at least once a month. Blood pressure screenings are available at these locations and times:

       Call the doctor if your blood pressure is above 150/90 or below 100/60.

    3. This drug *may* cause some of the following side effects in some people who take it. Not everyone will have them, but you may

experience one or more. Call the doctor if you experience any of those marked with a double asterisk (**).

drowsiness (call only if it continues after you have been taking the drug for two weeks)
headache
fever (call only if it is higher than 101 degrees)
weakness
dizziness, especially when arising from a chair or bed (call only if it is severe)
forgetfulness
numbness or tingling in arms or legs
nightmares
depression
facial paralysis
stuffy nose
angina (chest pain)
nausea and vomiting
constipation or diarrhea (call only if severe)
dry mouth
sore tongue (may also be black)
breast enlargement
sexual problems
muscle aches
dark urine

4. Call the doctor if you experience any additional symptoms not listed here after you begin taking your medication.

5. Do not drive a car or operate machinery if you get drowsy during the first two weeks of treatment.

Methyldopa Aldomet, Dopamet,* Mediment-250,*

Methyldopate HCl Aldomet Hydrochloride

Classification   Antihypertensive, depresses sympathetic nervous system.

Remarks   Methyldopa is an antihypertensive that causes little change in cardiac output. Note: Methyldopa is a component of Aldoril (see Appendix 3).

Action/ Kinetics   Primary mechanism thought to be that the active metabolic, alpha-methyl-norepinephrine lowers BP by stimulating central inhibitory alpha-adrenergic receptors, false neurotransmission, and/or reduction of plasma renin. **PO: Onset:** 7–12 hr. **Duration:** 12–24 hr. All effects terminated within 48 hr. Absorption is variable. **IV: Onset,** 4–6 hr. **Duration:** 10–16 hr. 70% of drug excreted in urine. **Full therapeutic effect:** 1–4 days.

Uses   Moderate to severe hypertension. Particularly useful for patients with impaired renal function, renal hypertension, resistant cases of hypertension complicated by stroke, coronary artery diseases, or nitrogen retention, and for hypertensive crises (parenterally).

Contra-   Sensitivity to drug, labile and mild hypertension,
indications   pregnancy, active hepatic disease, or pheochromocytoma. Use with caution in patients with history of liver disease.

Untoward   Sedation (tends to disappear with use), vertigo,
Reactions   headache, asthenia and weakness, orthostatic hypotension, syncope, aggravation of angina pectoris, paradoxical pressor response, sodium retention, edema, anemia, or fever (during initial weeks of therapy).
        Rare side effects include jaundice, bradycardia, nasal stuffiness, dry mouth, GI symptoms, "black tongue," breast enlargement, lactation, impotence, skin rash, mild arthralgia, myalgia, paresthesias, parkinsonism, and psychic disturbances. Affects Coombs' test—which may be indicative of hemolytic anemia.
        Many of these untoward reactions are dose related and disappear with continued use of the drug.

Drug
Interactions

Interactant	Interaction
Amphetamines	↓ Hypotensive effect of methyldopa by ↑ sympathetic activity
Anesthetics, general	Additive hypotension
Antidepressants, tricyclic	Tricyclic antidepressants may block hypotensive effect of methyldopa
Amitriptyline	
Nortriptyline	
Barbiturates	↓ Hypotensive effect of methyldopa by ↑ breakdown by liver

Ephedrine	Action of ephedrine ↓ in methyldopa-treated patients
Furazolidone (Furoxone)	Additive hypotensive effect
Haloperidol	Methyldopa ↑ toxic effects of haloperidol
Levodopa	Additive hypotensive effect
Lithium	↑ Possibility of lithium toxicity
Levodopa	Methyldopa inhibits effect of levodopa
Methotrimeprazine (Levoprome)	Additive hypotensive effect
MAO inhibitors Pargyline (Eutonyl) Tranylcypromine (Parnate)	May reverse hypotensive effect of methyldopa and cause headache and hallucinations
Norepinephrine (Levophed)	Magnitude and duration of pressor response to norepinephrine ↑ in patients receiving methyldopa
Phenothiazines	Additive hypotensive effect
Procarbazine (Matulane)	Additive hypotensive effect
Propranolol (Inderal)	Additive hypotensive effect
Quinidine	Additive hypotensive effect
Thiazide diuretics	Additive hypotensive effect
Tolbutamide	↑ Hypoglycemia due to ↓ breakdown by liver
Thioxanthines	Additive hypotensive effect
Vasodilator drugs Isoxsuprine (Vasoldilan) Nicotinyl alcohol (Roniacol) Nylidrin (Arlidin)	Additive hypotensive effect

Laboratory Test Interference False + or ↑ : Alkaline phosphatase, bilirubin, BUN, BSP, cephalin flocculation, creatinine, SGOT, SGPT, uric acid, Coombs' test, prothrombin time. Positive lupus erythematosis (LE) cell preparation and antinuclear antibodies.

Dosage *Methyldopa,* **PO: initial:** 250 mg b.i.d.–t.i.d. for 2 days. Adjust dose every 2 days. If increased, start with evening dose. **Usual maintenance:** 0.5–2.0 gm daily in divided doses; **maximum:** 3 gm daily. Transfer to and from other antihypertensive agents should occur gradually, with initial dose of methyldopa not exceeding 500 mg. *Remarks:* Do not use combination medication to initiate therapy. **Pediatric: Initial,** 10 mg/kg daily, adjusting maintenance to a maximum of 65 mg/kg. *Methyldopate HC1:* **IV infusion,** 250–500 mg q 6 hr; **maximum:** 1 gm q 6 hr for *hypertensive crisis.* Switch to oral methyldopa, at same dosage level, when blood pressure is brought under control. **Pediatric:** 20–40 mg/kg q 6 hr; **maximum:** 65 mg/kg up to maximum of 3 gm daily.

Nursing Implications

1. Ascertain that hematologic, liver function, and a Coombs' test are done before initiation of therapy. Periodic tests should be performed throughout therapy.
2. If the patient needs a blood transfusion, ascertain that both direct and indirect Coombs' tests are done. If the indirect as well as the direct Coombs' tests are positive, anticipate consultation with a blood transfusion specialist.
3. *Assess*
   a. for signs of tolerance which may occur during the second or third month of therapy.
   b. weight daily and observe carefully for edema.
   c. intake and output, observing particularly for reduced urine volume.
4. *Teach patient and/or family*
   a. that patient should rise from bed slowly and should dangle feet from edge of bed to prevent dizziness and fainting. Adjusting dosage may prevent morning hypotension.
   b. sedation may occur when therapy is first started, but that it disappears once the maintenance dose is established.
   c. that in rare cases methyldopa may darken urine or turn it blue, but that this reaction is not harmful.
   d. to inform anesthesiologist that patient is on methyldopa, if surgery is required.
   e. to withhold drug and report to doctor tiredness, fever, or yellowing of skin and whites of eyes.

    f. to inform doctor that patient is on methyldopa if he
       requires a transfusion, because the drug induces a
       positive Coombs' test.

These descriptions are so different because they have fundamentally different *purposes* and *audiences*. Although they share a common general goal—to communicate necessary information regarding Aldomet to the reader—the different forms result principally from important differences in *knowledge, attitudes,* and *needs* of the intended readers. In the case of the technical description, the writer assumes a health care professional who has extensive knowledge of technical vocabulary, understands the necessity of the medication, presumably is favorably disposed toward using the drug therapeutically, and requires detailed information concerning its pharmacologic effects. The handout for patients, on the other hand, assumes quite a different audience: someone whose knowledge is limited, who may not understand the need for taking the medication precisely as described, who may be fearful, and whose health (and perhaps life) depends upon taking it as prescribed and reporting potentially significant side effects.

The writer of the patient information sheet had to balance two conflicting factors: the need to provide enough information about the drug to be sure that the patient is adequately informed and the need to avoid language that is too technical or that might trigger psychosomatic side effects. Thus, the central nervous system effects from the *Handbook* have been translated into language easily understood by most patients. And the problems of reduced libido and impotence have been phrased generally as "sexual problems" to avoid suggestions that might become self-fulfilling prophecies. Different *audiences, needs,* and *goals* all must be taken into account when we think about how to communicate effectively.

WRITING READER-BASED PROSE

Your most effective writing will look beyond the simple question of "what do I want to say?" Your thoughts alone, no matter how clearly you express them, are not enough for effective communication. Only when you combine three elements—topic, purpose, and audience—can you create a message that will convey your meaning powerfully and effectively to the reader. Your topic will usually leave you little room for flexibility. After all, you usually do not have the option of writing about something other than the issue at hand, whether it is a change in the vacation schedule, a request for an increased budget, a personnel problem, or a letter of congratulation.

In practice, then, what makes some communication more effective is a thoughtful blending of *purpose* and *audience*. Decide why you are writing and what you want to achieve. Then analyze your audience. When you successfully match your own goals to the needs and attitudes of your audience, you will have prepared the most effective communication possible. In the following chapters, we will discuss some specific ways of achieving that goal.

2

Getting Started

Once you have decided to write reader-based prose, you need to consider three aspects of your situation (what writing theorists call the *rhetorical situation*). The three elements you need to think about are:

- Your *purpose* in writing
- The *reader* (or readers) of your document
- How to present *yourself* to your readers

Only when you have carefully considered all of these can you design a document that will do what you want it to do.

YOUR PURPOSE

A writer may have many purposes in writing: to entertain, to express creativity, to ventilate emotion, and so on. However, most of the writing you face on the job will be designed to achieve one of these ends:

- To *inform* your readers of something they need to know
- To *persuade* them to do something you want them to do

Think carefully about precisely what you want your readers to do with the document you are writing. Purposes can be complex, depending upon what you want to convey, and labelling your purpose as either informing *or* persuading is somewhat misleading. You may have more than one purpose—to inform *and* to persuade, for example. Consider this example. As a director of nursing services, you have been told that diagnosis related groups (DRGs) are having an adverse effect on the budget of the entire hospital. Nursing has been affected by a 10% reduction in your budget for the next fiscal year, which will mean an actual reduction of perhaps 20% when proposed salary increases are taken into account. After much thought, you have decided to institute this decrease in the form of an across-the-board cut equally distributed among all nursing services. You are about to write the memo explaining your decision to all your nurse managers.

Upon first consideration, your goal seems simple: all you want to do is inform supervisors, head nurses, and other managers of your decision. But think a minute; the situation is more complex than it might seem. (Isn't that always the case for nurse managers?) Although you want to inform, you also want the readers of your memo to understand why you have had to do what you've done—that it was the right thing to do under the circumstances. That is, you want to *persuade* as well. We're not suggesting that you offer a detailed rationale for every decision you make. You'd spend all your time explaining. But wise managers seek the support and understanding of subordinates whenever possible. Some administrators believe that employees will simply do what they're told. That's probably true. Nevertheless, it's better if they understand and agree rather than having to be forced. Persuasion is nearly always more effective than coercion.

Sometimes, of course, your audience is unlikely to agree with what you have to say. In such cases, you may never be able to convince them that your action is correct or desirable. But you might be able to show that it's necessary, or at least that you've considered their point of view before making your decision. Even such limited persuasion—that you're reasonable rather than arbitrary—is worth seeking.

YOUR READER

You can write reader-based prose only if you have a clear understanding of the receiver of your communication—your reader. A few minutes' thought about the characteristics of your reader *before* you begin to write will usually pay off in more effective writing. In particular, you will want to assess what your reader feels and what he or she knows about you and your topic. Ask yourself these general questions. Is my reader:

- Interested or uninterested in what I have to say?
- Likely to be pleased or displeased?
- Knowledgeable or ignorant of my subject?
- Sympathetic or hostile toward me? toward my topic?

It should be clear that readers who are interested, pleased, knowledgeable, and sympathetic will be much easier to convince than those who are not. On the other hand, writers have to work very hard to achieve their goals with readers who are bored, unhappy, ignorant, and hostile. Sometimes, our writing will have more than one kind of reader, especially if we write to a large audience. The patient information sheet in Chapter 1, for example, is addressed primarily to patients, but it may also be read (and judged) by other health care professionals, including nurses, physicians, and pharmacists. Devote most attention to the characteristics of your primary audience, but also consider the others who will read it.

STATEMENT OF PURPOSE AND AUDIENCE (SoPA)

A helpful way to organize your thoughts about purpose and audience is a form such as that shown in Figure 2.1.

This form directs your attention to some of the important points to consider about any document you may need to write. Of course, some aspects of the form will be less applicable to some tasks, and no single document is likely to require you to fill out the form completely. But if you take it step by step, you will have a convenient summary of your responses to these important questions:

- What (in general) is the message I want to convey?
- Why am I writing this document?

STATEMENT OF PURPOSE AND AUDIENCE

SCOPE: What is your topic? Where did you go to get your information?

_____

_____

_____

_____

PURPOSES: What purposes will your document serve?

_____

_____

_____

_____

AUDIENCES: Who will read your document? Who else is concerned about what your document is like?

The *primary* readers who are important to you are:

1. _____   2. _____

The *secondary* readers who are also important to you are:

1. _____   2. _____

3. _____   4. _____

Some important characteristics of the *primary* audience that might affect how you write the document are:

1. _____

2. _____

3. _____

4. _____

For the *secondary* audiences, you should be concerned about these points:

Audience _____   Concerns _____

_____

Audience _____   Concerns _____

_____

Audience _____   Concerns _____

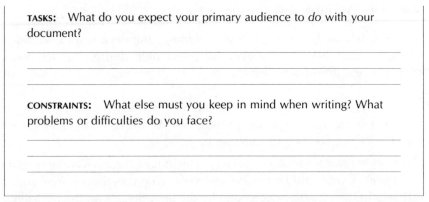

TASKS: What do you expect your primary audience to *do* with your document?

_____

_____

CONSTRAINTS: What else must you keep in mind when writing? What problems or difficulties do you face?

_____

_____

_____

Figure 2.1. Statement of purpose and audience. (Adapted from Dixie Goswami et al., *Writing in the Professions,* 1981. This material is reprinted by permission from the Document Design Center, American Institutes for Research.)

- Who will read it, and what do I know about them?
- What do I expect the readers to do with the document?
- What constraints must I keep in mind?

Here are some points to consider as you complete each portion of the SoPA form.

What (in General) is the Message I Want to Convey?

Consider what it is that you need (or must) do. Some common examples might be:

- A memo to the director of nursing requesting permission to hire an additional staff person
- A brochure explaining emergency room procedures to patients
- A description of a proposed research study
- A textbook for nurse managers on how to write clear, useful documents

Why Am I Writing This Document?

Here you will analyze your *purposes* in writing your document. In addition to the example discussed above, these may help clarify what we mean by purposes. If you are writing:

> *A letter applying for a job,* your ultimate purpose is probably to get the job, but the immediate purpose is to be selected for an interview. The clever writer will consider both.
>
> *A memo summmarizing a meeting,* you might have a variety of purposes. One might be to have everyone who was there see on paper what you think they agreed to before anyone acts on the decisions. Another purpose might be to leave a written record in the file for future reference.
>
> *Policies or procedures,* you usually want to write clear instructions to help staff operate equipment or perform procedures easily and correctly. (As we will discuss in Chapter 6, there are important differences between the purposes of policies and the purposes of procedures. That's why they should be written differently.)

Who Will Read It?

This question addresses the matter of audience—or, more precisely in most cases, *audiences* who will read your document. To grasp how important an understanding of audience can be, consider this situation. Imagine that you have had a particularly rough day, one of those in which everything possible has gone wrong. At the end of the day, you get to the parking lot and discover that your car has a flat tire—and it's raining. How would you express yourself about the day if you were telling your best friend? Your father? Your daughter? Your minister? Chances are that you would communicate very differently to each of these people. Yet your subject would be the same and so would your essential purpose. The variations in each communication would result from differences among your audiences and your relationship to them.

Writing on the job involves similar distinctions. Depending upon your topic and purpose, you may write to people inside or outside your organization, knowledgeable or ignorant of your topic, sympathetic or hostile to you, and so on. Even within your organization, various audiences may need to be addressed differently: hospital administrators and physicians don't necessarily use the same vocabulary.

One of the most difficult tasks is addressing *multiple audiences* in one document that will be read by (and must meet the needs of) many groups. A writer designing an informed consent form for a surgical procedure, for example, would consider these audiences and needs:

- The patient (or patient's family), who should be able to understand the form in order to supply consent that is truly informed
- The practitioner, who seeks to limit potential liability
- The hospital, which also seeks to limit liability, but whose interests are not the same as the practitioner's

In cases such as this, you may find it impossible to design a document that will address all audiences' needs equally well. To see that this is so, just examine the next informed consent form you see. Whose needs are principally served, whose neglected?

Often, though, you *can* accommodate the needs of multiple audiences in a single document if you plan carefully. In many personnel actions, especially terminations, managers must pay attention to the fact that a variety of people may read a document and put it to different uses: the person being fired, the personnel office, and, potentially at least, lawyers, judges, and jurors. To ignore these secondary audiences is to invite disaster.

What Do I Expect Readers to Do with My Document?

You should be sensitive not only to *who* your audience is, but also to *how* readers will *use* the document. Depending on what you're writing, readers may need to

- Read to understand
- Read to locate information
- Read to act immediately (put something together, use a new procedure)
- Read and answer questions to fill out a form

Your reader's task can be made more or less difficult by the way you organize and present your material.

What Constraints Must I Keep in Mind?

Nearly all writing tasks include constraints imposed by yourself, by outsiders, or by the situation. The most obvious of these are

- Deadline
- Length
- Budget
- Resources (especially other people) that you may be able to draw upon for help

Keeping in mind the constraints you must face, and devising strategies to deal with them, will help you create a document that is most effective.

PRESENTING YOURSELF

Some of the writing that nurses do is (or ought to be) completely objective, but most nurse managers have gone beyond the time when their writing is confined largely to charting and care plans. As we have said earlier, much of the writing that any manager does is *persuasive,* and an important part of persuasion is how the reader reacts to the writer. So we urge you to think carefully about the way you present yourself to your reader.

Consider the characteristics you value in the people you work with and for: if you're like most of us, you prefer those who are fair, reasonable, objective, sensitive, sympathetic, friendly, warm, and so on. If you have reason to trust someone and to believe that he has done his homework carefully, you are more likely to accept what he says willingly. On the other hand, if you believe he's undependable, mean-spirited, and biased, you'll be less inclined to go along with what he says—regardless of the subject. The same thing with your relationship to your reader. If she believes that you're honest, fair, reasonable, and sympathetic, she's far more likely to be persuaded by your writing than if she does not believe this. Even when your message will be unwelcome, you can lower resistance to it by the way you come across as a writer. If you sound arrogant and dictatorial, you will automatically arouse unnecessary resistance to your message. If you make mistakes in facts, spelling, or punctuation, readers who recognize those facts will make certain assumptions about you that will affect the way they respond to your message.

Take care, therefore, to pay attention to the details of your writing. In addition to making sure that the details and mechanics are correct, consider carefully what *tone* you want to use. Your readers, like all of us, want to believe that they're taken seriously as human beings, that their work and views are valued, that they're being treated fairly, and that other people care about them. The more you can project these characteristics in your writing, the more effective it is likely to be.

To a certain extent, this means allowing your real personality to come through in your writing, and we encourage you to develop a writing style that reflects your personality. If you are enthusiastic and happy most of the time, don't feel compelled to adopt a writing style that is formal and excessively serious. You have probably reached your management position because you *do* have the sort of personality that makes an effective manager. Let that personality show through in your writing.

Imagine that you have applied for the position of assistant director of nursing at your hospital. After an extensive evaluation process, you became one of three finalists, but you have not yet heard what decision was made. Which of these letters would you rather receive?

Dear Ms. Koslonski:

The position of assistant director of nursing has now been filled, and you have not been selected. This is in no way a reflection on your qualifications, and your application received serious consideration. Thank you very much for applying. I wish you the best of luck in your career here at Grasmere State Hospital.

Sincerely,

E. Louise Wardle, R.N., M.S.N
Director of Nursing

Dear Marlene:

As you may know, we have now selected another candidate as assistant director of nursing. Although I'm sure you are disappointed, perhaps you will take some comfort from the fact that you made the final three out of a very strong group of applicants.

Mr. Heinlen and I were particularly impressed by the way you have performed as the clinical specialist in the oncology unit. Your work with the family support groups and the hospice program have made real differences in the lives of patients and their families. Because of your energy, creativity, and sensitivity, you were a strong candidate for the position. I'm sure you will continue to provide important leadership in nursing here at Grasmere.

                              Sincerely,

                              Louise Wardle

The first letter is stiff, formal, and distant. Why would Wardle use her degrees and title when writing to someone who presumably knows her well? The second letter is much more effective, not only because it is reader-centered, but also because the director of nursing allows herself to come across in the letter as a sensitive human being who has just had to make a difficult decision about her new assistant director. In the second letter, the writer offers words of encouragement and praise that, while not excessive, reveal to the recipient that the writer values her as a nurse and cares about her feelings. Such a letter takes only a bit longer to write and will pay dividends in good will and positive feelings.

MAKE A PLAN

Most inexperienced writers underestimate the importance of planning *before* writing. Writing teachers have known for years that the steps taken before writing can be the most important in generating an effective document. Some of the things we have already mentioned are important steps in the prewriting process—in particular the analysis of purpose and audience discussed earlier in this chapter. Careful thought about why you're writing and to whom will help you determine a strategy that will be effective with your topic and audience. But that still leaves many important decisions to be made—about format, organization, and so on.

The most basic of these is to decide what kind of structure to use for your document. Certain decisions in this regard may well be dictated by your reasons for writing: do you face a long budget report or a short informal memo to someone in the organization? For the latter, organizational problems are often minimal, especially if your topic is simple and your intended message short. But longer documents require more thought. Even a one-page letter may very well involve two or three subtopics, and you must determine the most effective order, what sort of explanation is required, how much detail, and so on.

One of the best techniques for organizing your thoughts is the one with which you are probably the most familiar: the outline. You may recall one of your teachers insisting upon certain rules about outlines: never use an A without a B, progress from capital letters with roman numerals down to lower case letters with arabic numerals, use parentheses to show smaller subdivisions. If you're like us, you probably thought outlining was an elaborate science unto itself, one to be mastered only after intensive study.

Our advice now is to forget all those rules. Although they are logical and helpful in developing skills in analysis and subdivision, they're not important to you as you prewrite. So use any sort of outlining that makes sense to you and that you're comfortable with. Your aim in outlining is not to satisfy some prickly pedagogue, but help you organize your thoughts. They're yours, so you can work with them any way you please. Your aim is simply to arrange your thoughts so you can control them as you draft your document. Here's an example—the outline we devised for this chapter up to this point:

II. Getting Started
　　A. Define the Rhetorical Problem and Understand Your Goals
　　　　1. Your purpose
　　　　　　a. inform
　　　　　　b. persuade

    2. Your reader
       a. interested or uninterested?
       b. pleased or displeased?
       c. knowledgeable or ignorant?
       d. sympathetic or hostile?
    3. Statement of purpose and audience
    4. Presenting yourself
  B. Make a Plan
    1. Outlining

The outline has served for us as a sort of skeleton to organize our ideas into a sequence that we could flesh out as we wrote. You can do the same. Make an outline that is long or short, as detailed or sketchy, as orderly or messy as you like. No one will ever see it, but if you do it well, everyone will be able to follow what you write.

WHAT TO DO WHEN YOU CAN'T GET STARTED

One of the most fearsome sights to anyone who has a deadline is the icy whiteness of a blank sheet of paper. Even experienced writers constantly find real difficulty in getting started. Many times, the techniques we've already discussed will help get the juices flowing, for the Statement of Purpose and Audience and your outline will push you in the right direction. Other times, however, you remain blocked: the words just won't come. What can you do? If you have enough time, you can sometimes just wait things out; eventually the spirit will probably move you. But too often we don't have the luxury of waiting. The new procedure must be sent out now. The budget report is due at the end of the month. The publisher wants the manuscript by January 1. In short, these are times when we must write *now*.

Over the years, terrified writers like you (and us) have found some ways of overcoming writer's block. Not all of them work for everyone, but most of them are helpful for some people sometimes. Try one of these. If it doesn't work, try another.

- Free writing
- Making lists
- R & R with percolation

Chances are that one of these will help you limber up your brain and begin to say what you want to say.

Free Writing

Free writing as a way of discovering ideas grows out of an unusual theory called *automatic writing*. This idea, which derives loosely from Freud's theory of the unconscious, is an effort to cause a writer's subconscious thoughts to emerge on paper. The rationale was that if people could force themselves to keep writing at a steady pace, writing down whatever popped into their minds, no matter how silly or disconnected it seemed, their subconscious ideas would begin to pour forth. The originator hoped that a kind of poetry or important art form would result. With us, as with some people, the results are most often curious rather than artistic, but the process does seem to limber up the mind in some way, allowing ideas to emerge. Try it, following these guidelines:

1. Write about whatever comes to mind as you think about your topic. Just relax and let your ideas flow, no matter how silly or unusual they maybe.

2. Once you begin, do not stop writing *for a full five minutes.* Don't even pause. The five minutes will seem like a much longer time. Write at a steady, even pace.

3. If you run out of ideas, keep writing the last word over and over until a new thought pops up. One will.

4. Don't worry about spelling, punctuation, or even making sense. Feel free to jump from one thought to another. You can write in sentences, phrases, or even unrelated words. Remember, you're writing only for yourself.

5. When you have finished, review what you have written. Most likely, you'll find something that will help generate your document.

Making Lists

This technique allows you to generate lists of words, concepts, or topics which you will later edit and organize. The simplest might be lists of *pro* and *con* related to your topic. Or you might use the "journalists' questions": who, what, when, where, how, why. Decide what sort of structure suggests itself, create your headings on a blank piece of paper, and you're off. Once again, don't worry about producing complete sentences or even complete phrases—single words will do. Your aim is simply to get as many ideas as possible on paper; later, you can read your lists and see what concepts and patterns emerge. We often begin with lists, then move to the outline as a second stage of organization.

R & R With Percolation

Sometimes even the techniques we've described above won't be enough. Your ideas just won't flow, things won't come together. In those cases, we recommend that you simply walk away from your material for a while. Try rest and recreation (R & R). If you have tried outlining, free writing, and making lists and you still don't seem ready to write, go off and do something else. Even if you can't get R & R, while you're working at some other task, the materials you've been thinking about will be bubbling in your head, and it may be easier to write when you get back to it than it was before. This doesn't always work, but if you have the luxury of letting your task lie fallow for a time, it's worth trying.

3

Reviewing and Editing

Up to this point, we have emphasized how to go about planning your document and beginning to get it on paper. Once you begin to write, however, you need to consider other matters: what kind of language do I want to use to achieve a particular purpose with a particular audience? Shall I use big words or small? Should I use a technical vocabulary or will jargon interfere with my purpose? How will the language I use reflect upon me? What language will communicate my message clearly and forcefully? These considerations become most important *after* you have written your first draft, as you begin to refine your work through the editing process. But even if you don't always have time to edit your work completely, the information we cover in this chapter should help you become aware of some of the ways language affects your readers.

LEVELS OF LANGUAGE

The question "what word should I use?" can be difficult. *Contemplate* and *think* are both good, useful words, but which one you choose to use depends upon what style you have decided to adopt for your document.

Questions about what sort of word to use arise because there are different varieties of English and because these varieties don't fit equally well into every rhetorical (and social) occasion. What would be clear to a group of English professors might baffle an audience of high school students. Language that would be natural and appropriate in conversation among good friends isn't always suitable in the hospital newsletter. Imagine, for example, that you have just had a long, fruitless discussion with an administrator whose stupidity has left you frustrated and angry. How would you relate the experience and your feelings to these audiences?: your best friend, your parents, your six-year old nephew, and the hospital chaplain. If you're like most people, you would choose very different words for each person. "Good English" isn't just arbitrarily good. It's good because it's right for the occasion, the purpose, and the audience.

Formal English

Formal English sounds to most people excessively elevated, like a sermon or a graduation speech. It is the language sometimes used in textbooks for advanced students or articles written by professors for other professors. Here is an example taken from a book on the history of Christianity:

> Thus the reform movement in France had never been buttressed by the salient force of xenophobia and nationalism, and that was the principal reason why it had never become the majority. Instead, the essential conflict was fought out in the seventeenth century within the French Catholic Church itself, with the puritanical Jansenists representing moral and doctrinal reform, the Jesuits and the crown standing for traditional Catholic authority, and an entirely secular third force pressing the claims of reason.

The vocabulary of formal English includes words seldom used in ordinary conversation (*buttressed, salient, xenophobia*) and a high proportion of nouns. Moreover, it tends to use long, involved sentences (as in the second sentence above). Formal English can be both elegant and precise, as with this sample, but it can also be difficult to follow or, for someone who doesn't share the vocabulary, impossible to understand.

If you ever set out to write in the formal style, you run some significant risks. Unless you control it carefully, it may end up sounding unintentionally funny, or so self-conscious that it obscures your message.

The bad imitations of formal language that we all encounter seem to derive principally from one of two motives. The writer desires either to obfuscate and confuse or to impress with ponderous bulk and complexity. In the hands of all but a few sensitive writers, the formal style frequently falls flat. Unless you have a very clear reason for using formal language, we recommend that you avoid it.

Informal English

At the other end of the spectrum of written language we encounter informal English, the kind of language we use naturally in letters to close friends and family members, diaries and journals, and other forms of close, intimate expression. In some ways, informal written English suggests common patterns of speech—using slang words, shoptalk, abbreviated forms ("I bet he'll be sorry" rather than "I'll bet that he will be sorry").

In general, you will probably want to avoid informal English as well as elaborately formal English. Although you will perhaps encounter occasions when an informal note will be most appropriate, readers will often be put off by language that they consider too slangy or colloquial. Informal English isn't bad, but it will often be inappropriate to your audience and occasion. With both formal and informal English, we suggest this guideline: avoid them unless you have clear reason for using them.

General English

General English occupies the broad middle ground between the formal and the informal. It's the variety of standard English that the majority of educated writers write and expect to read. Because your readers will expect to encounter it most of the time, you run risks if you deviate too far from the middle. Although general English can accommodate *whacko, insane,* and *mentally unbalanced,* you're usually safest choosing language that is less slangy than *wacko* and less stuffy than *mentally unbalanced. Insane* or perhaps *crazy* would usually be the word to use. You should feel free to vary your word choice, of course, when you seek a specific effect: surprise, humor, erudition. But in general, you should seek a middle-of-the-road level of language. General English is best because it will reach more people more consistently than either formal or informal English. It's the kind of language we're using throughout this book, though we frequently use informal features and, less frequently, formal language. This is not to suggest that you should cultivate a bland, "average" writing style. In fact, your writing should reflect your personality. (Perhaps the reason some writing sounds stuffy is that it was written by stuffy people.) We urge you to seek a tone and style of writing that conveys a sense of who you are and what you're like. But we think you'll agree that it's probably not useful to sound like a nut or a fuddy-duddy, even if that's what you are.

TONE AND STYLE

One effect of a particular level of language is that it will help create a *tone*. When we speak of the tone of a document, we mean something like what is meant by the phrase "tone of voice." Regardless of the message a speaker means to convey, she can deliver it in a variety of ways: sympathetically, sarcastically, sadly, temperamentally. The writer, too, can control tone through choice of detail, word choice, word order, sentence length, and so on.

In every document the writer consciously or unconsciously reveals something about himself or herself. Here are two examples, both from the prefaces to recently published textbooks.

> The effective nurse is portrayed as able to lead and to manage. Leadership and management are presented as a learned process that can become habitual with practice. To be successful a leader must have followers. The nurse leader earns the right to direct others within formal or informal situations. Managers, on the other hand, are appointed to their positions and may or may not possess leadership qualities. Effective nurses acquire skill as leaders and managers, thereby becoming able to function in the health care delivery system with assurance, knowing they are well equipped for their roles.

> What have you written lately? Your immediate response may be, "Nothing. I'm not a writer," but think again. You have almost surely held a pen, pencil,

or crayon in your hand in the last forty-eight hours and written something. Or perhaps, like me, you do most of your writing at the typewriter. If you really think about your activities for the last few days, they probably included at least two or three of these:

- A check to pay a bill
- A grocery list
- An excused absence note for a son or daughter
- Lecture notes in a college class
- A memo to a coworker about a job to be done
- A thank you note
- A limerick about someone you dislike
- A note to your wife, husband, or roommate to explain why you would be coming home late

Both paragraphs are written in approximately the same level of general English, yet they are significantly different in tone. The first makes no mention of either writer or reader (and therefore is not reader-centered). When material "is portrayed" or concepts "are presented," we want to know *who* is portraying or presenting this information, but the paragraph gives no sense of a person writing to other people. Although the distinction between a leader and a manager may be important for nursing administrators, it is delivered in dull and lifeless prose.

The second paragraph, on the other hand, is lively and much more interesting, partly because the writer understands the importance of reader-centered writing. This paragraph is written to real readers with feelings and needs. They think they don't write and probably consider writing as foreign and threatening. They need comfort and reassurance, and the tone of the passage offers that. Most of us would be relieved to encounter a writer who shares some of our problems, has thought about them carefully, and writes to us as one human to another. If you had to read 75 pages in the next two hours, would you rather read the first book or the second? Subject matter aside, almost all of us would choose the second. It's clearer, more accessible, more human, more *interesting*.

Presenting Yourself

One effect of tone is to convey to the reader a sense of the writer. What sort of person is writing this? Is he intelligent, careful, sensitive, sympathetic? Does she care about my position? Is she fair? Or is he pushy and dictatorial, unsympathetic, sloppy, stupid? Even matters as simple as correct spelling and punctuation will influence your reader. How would this sentence affect you if you read it in a letter?

> *I seen him yesterday after work.*

The second word in the sentence, of course, should be *saw,* and readers who detect the error would be likely to conclude one of two things. Either the writer doesn't know the correct form (and therefore lacks important knowledge—how smart is she?) or didn't take the time to proofread the letter (and is therefore careless—is he always this sloppy? Will he make mistakes with more important things as well?). In either case, the reader has begun to make judgments about the writer.

Writing nearly four centuries before the birth of Christ, Aristotle described the effect of personality on the process of communication. In his *Rhetoric,* he wrote of speaker and hearer, but what he said pertains to writer and reader as well.

> But since the art of speech aims at producing certain judgments. . .the speaker must not only look at his words, to see they are cogent and convincing, he must also present himself as a certain type of person and put those who judge him in a certain frame of mind. . . .For it makes all the difference to men's opinions whether they feel friendly or hostile, irritated or indulgent. . . .To carry conviction, a speaker needs three qualitites—for there are three things that convince us, apart from actual proof—good sense, good character, and good will towards hearers.

We can help determine the personality we project in our documents by:

- Carefully avoiding errors
- Being reasonable in our assumptions and requests
- Showing an awareness of the other person's position

- Allowing our own individuality to be expressed in our writing
- Being as positive and courteous as the occasion will allow

Jargon

In one sense, *jargon* means shoptalk, the words professionals use when speaking to one another about their work. Technical terms have technical uses, and you need not apologize for using them if the technical meaning is the one you must have. Sometimes, too, jargon can offer a kind of shorthand communication, encompassing a long, technical process or meaning into one term. This, too, is valuable because it helps us communicate clearly and economically.

On the other hand, *jargon* also means fuzzy, pretentious language—wordiness, overuse of "big" abstract words, and words which inflate but add no meaning. This meaning includes the overuse of *buzz words* and *gobbledygook:* current examples include *impact, dialogue* (as a verb), *parameters, interface* (as a verb), and others. Much current jargon comes (often inappropriately) from the language of the social sciences, especially psychology and sociology. For evidence of its impact on the vocabulary of nursing, consider these sentences, which we collected by going to the library, pulling from the shelf an introduction to nursing textbook, and leafing randomly through its pages.

In developing the adaptation concept of nursing certain classes of relevant contextual stimuli are being identified for certain circumstances.

Fatigue and insomnia are the major problems noted with deficits in the need for rest. Nursing interventions indicated when these problems are identified include the manipulation of the stimuli that are causing or contributing to the maladaptive behavior noted.

Once the adaptive or maladaptive nutritional behaviors have been made and the problem cited or a nursing diagnosis made, client goals (adaptive behaviors) and nursing interventions that manipulate the validated stimuli can be formulated.

Sick role failure occurs when there is an absence of feelings or expressive behaviors and/or a lack of action or instrumental behaviors appropriate to the patient's stage of illness and his position on the health/illness continuum.

These sentences are not, of course, absolutely typical of the kind of writing nurses do. But the fact that we could locate them so easily—quite literally in just a few minutes of leafing through a book chosen at random—confirms our sense that the writing of many nurses (like other professionals) employs jargon frequently and often indiscriminately. Jargon does not make for writing that is incomprehensible, at least not always, but it often impedes the transfer of meaning from writer to reader. In most of the examples we've just cited, you will probably be able to figure out what the writer is seeking to say. But in every sentence, we think, much of the jargon obscures rather than conveys what the writer has to say.

So why do nurses use jargon? Sometimes it's just habit; such words are all around us, and we may use them without much thought. Another reason is as a defense: nurses who worry about sounding professional enough may feel the need to inflate their language in the hope that they will be taken seriously by other health care professionals. They seem to share this characteristic with other professional groups. Educators and social scientists, in particular, seem to feel the need to beef up their language, to make it sound objective, scientific, profound. But more often than not, we think, other professionals who read such inflated prose are likely to find it confusing or—at its worst—unintentionally funny.

On other occasions, nurses may fear that a good idea simply expressed won't be recognized as a good idea. So they translate plain words into multisyllabic, sesquipedalian wonders that may cow the reader into submission. ("Sesquipedalian," in case your dictionary is not at hand, means literally "a foot and a half long"; it has come to mean "of or pertaining to long words." We used it to illustrate what we mean about long words getting in the way of communication rather than helping it.) Much use of jargon, we suspect, comes from the feeling that writers won't be taken seriously unless they use big buzz words. Although this is an intuitive conclusion, a recent study confirms it for graduate students in business. The authors found that both graduate students and professors in MBA programs generally "respect big words and long sentences," and articles that were difficult to read were judged more competent than the same material presented in more accessible language (Lane N. Tracy and James A. Lee, "Acculturation of Business Students to Academic Values: Abstruseness as a Criterion of Competence," *Collegiate News & Views*, Vol. 38, No. 1 [Fall-Winter 1984], 37–41).

Big words and fancy jargon may, therefore, be functional with some audiences. The problem, of course, is that if readers are lost, confused, or exasperated by your language, you won't communicate anything at all. If you don't have anything to say, perhaps that's not bad. No one will discover your ignorance. But if you really do want to communicate something clearly and forcefully, without bamboozling the reader, we recommend that you avoid jargon (or "eschew obfuscation," as one wag phrased it).

Sexist Language

The growing movement toward equality of the sexes that has characterized the last 10 years has brought with it an increasing awareness of the ways language can reflect a bias against women—that is, *sexism.* Examples of usage that patronizes or denigrates women abound in English. *The little woman, the weaker sex, woman driver,* all suggest a negative view of women. The matter has become a very sensitive issue to many people, and effective writers ignore the issue at their peril.

What is the usual designation for the women who staff a physician's office? More often than not, we hear people speak of "Dr. Watson's *girls,"* yet if she had male assistants would they be called *boys?* Probably not, for to label grown men "boys" would be considered demeaning. To call adult women "girls" also demeans them, yet the practice is widespread. To many people, perhaps, such an example seems inoffensive, yet many others may find it objectionable (as we do). Therefore, unless you are certain that your readers will not object, you are wise to avoid any suggestion of sexism in your language. Frequent (or even occasional) use of such language will leave you open to the charge of being either sexist or insensitive, and neither is useful to the writer.

Yet the idea of sexism is still relatively new, and different groups have reached different stages of resentment against sex-biased language. It is difficult to know how far to go in ridding our language of the suggestion of sexism. The now-common title *Ms.* offers an alternative to the practice of designating a woman according to her marital status and offers a neutral equivalent to *Mr.* In many parts of the country, its use has become routine, but here where we live and write it is still relatively uncommon. This is but a simple indication of the difficulty of reacting to recent language change. To the women who use the title, *Ms.* suggests enlightenment and lack of bias. On the other hand, more conservative individuals may react differently, viewing someone who calls herself *Ms.* as somehow radical and perhaps threatening. Such is the power of language.

The point is that you must judge what steps you want (or need) to take in changing your own language. As we have so often stressed, intelligent writers make such decisions based upon the relationship among purpose, audience, and personality. With that in mind, we can offer some suggestions about how to deal with gender-biased language. The first step is to realize that language with sexist implications can originate in a number of different sources. The strategy for dealing with each varies.

BARBARISMS

These are usages that are so clearly inappropriate no sensible writer would use them: *broad, chick, tomato, typical female logic, typical male brutality, schoolgirl crush.* SOLUTION: avoid them entirely.

TITLES WITH INAPPROPRIATE IMPLICATIONS

Because of the changing nature of the world, many positions and occupations that were once nearly all-male or all-female have names that no longer fit: *stewardess, policeman, chairman.* In most cases, suitably neutral substitutions will occur: *stewardess* becomes *flight attendant, policeman* changes to *police officer,* and so on. But many of the titles ending with -*man* offer no such easy transformation. Most people tend to translate the -*man* into -*person,* but such a practice often creates words that clot sentences with their inelegant bulk. *Chairperson, weatherperson,* and the like offend the ear of many writers and should probably be avoided. Seek a neutral term that doesn't saddle you with a ponderous word: *head* for *chairman,* perhaps, or *meteorologist* for *weatherman. Male nurse* and *lady doctor*, of course, are easily dealt with: simply remove the unnecessary adjective.

Yet you cannot always find good substitutions, and you may sometimes be stuck with the inelegant but useful *-person*. What other construction comes to mind for alternatives to *spokesman, salesman,* or *layman?* In addition, one is faced with the question of what to do with other *man* words: *mankind, manmade, manhole*. Indeed, are these words sexist at all? The answer is that they are to some people and are not to others. You might seek substitute words that do not sound too out-of-the-way: *humanity* is a good substitute for *mankind*, and *synthetic* might serve for *man-made,* but which of us is happy with *personhole* for *manhole?*

SOLUTION: try to be sensitive to the problem. Recognize the effect of such vocabulary on certain people, then strike a balance between what your readers expect and your own sense of what is appropriate.

THE GENERIC "HE"

A central problem derives from the so-called *common gender*. What words should be used when we're discussing an indefinite person, a "one"? Traditionally, the pronoun has been male, not because the indefinite subject is always presumed to be male, but rather for the sake of convenience. For example:

Each *employee* should have *his* phone number on file.

According to the rules of grammar, the singular noun *employee* must take a singular pronoun. The fact that we choose to use *his*, the argument runs, does not mean that we believe all the employees are male. Indeed, we know better. It is simply a convention. The masculine pronoun designates not just men but all people of either sex.

Nevertheless, writers should understand that many people will object to this usage because it serves as a reminder of second-class citizenship for women. Therefore, you will probably want to consider alternatives to it. Some solutions that have been offered include using *he or she* (or *she or he* or *s/he*) consistently for common gender and treating singular words as plural *(Each employee should have their phone number on file)*. Yet each presents a problem. Continual repetition of *she or he* is ponderously monotonous, and most educated readers would object to violating good grammar to achieve verbal equality. Here are three general suggestions for dealing with the generic "he":

1. Use plurals to avoid the singular pronoun:

    All employees should have their phone numbers on file.

2. Show your awareness of the problem by using both *he* and *she* in your writing. You can add variety by combining this tactic with the occasional one of *he and she* or *she and he* (we have done both in this book).

3. Leave out the pronoun when it isn't required: not *Everone likes his bacon crisp* but *Everyone likes crisp bacon.*

All of these solutions are to some degree an imperfect compromise because we lack a consensus on how to handle common gender. But each of them has the merit of allowing you to present your ideas without making needless enemies among your readers.

EDITING FOR CLARITY AND FORCE

As you revise and reshape your documents, keep trying to make your sentences clear and forceful. In most cases, this means expressing yourself directly and economically. These guidelines will help you shape your sentences effectively.

Cut Out the Deadwood

Excessive words contribute nothing but clutter to your writing. Weed out the ones you don't need. They often lurk in phrases that come to mind as we're writing but can be eliminated upon revision. Sometimes they can be cut completely:

In [regards to] nursing theory, baccalaureate nurses seem better qualified [at this point in time].

Recent developments in [the field of] outpatient surgery have affected the way hospitals operate.

Ms. Jones was promoted because [of the fact that] she has the best qualifications.

On other occasions, we use a multiword phrase when one little word would do just as well:

	instead of
at the present time	now
at this point in time	now
during the time that	while
in the event that	if
in light of the fact that	because
prior to	before
subsequent to	after
upon the conclusion of	after

If you reread your drafts looking for such unnecessary words, you'll nearly always find them. When you do, strike them out.

Attack Flabby Words

At some point in our school years most of us learned that big words impressed our teachers more than little ones. The same thing often worked with our professors. Will it succeed with our bosses and colleagues too? Probably. So we use big words when little ones would work as well, often better. Some of the reasons may be similar to the reasons we use to much jargon: to impress, to be taken seriously, sometimes to obscure the fact that we don't have much to say. So we might end up writing:

Professors must endeavor to facilitate cognizance of the deleterious result of excessively sesquipedalian rhetorical structures.

or

Successful transplantation and bodily acceptance of the cardiac tissue depends upon administration of antirejection therapeutic modalities prior to and subsequent to the surgical procedure.

If you really want to communicate meaning to an audience, you'll seek words that are precise and to the point. Usually, given a choice between two words that mean the same thing, the shorter one will be better. Of course, sometimes you may need the long word to convey a precise meaning that you can't achieve with a little one. But too often we reach for the fancy word when the plain one will work just as well. And, being clearer, it's better. Here is a list of some common big words and their more direct equivalents:

Facilitate—help	Endeavor—try
Cognizant of—aware of	Implement—start, begin, carry out
Termination—end	
Impact on—affect (verb)	Dialogue—talk
Transpire—happen	Envisage—think, see
Parameters—borders, limits	Transmit—send
Utilize—use	Subsequent to—after

Others will no doubt occur to you. When you encounter such monsters, bear in mind the point we keep repeating: If you have a good reason for using the fancy word, do it. Otherwise, choose the one that is simple and clear.

Use Strong Verbs

One of the things that determines a clear, direct style is how we express action (which includes feeling, process, condition, etc.). The clearest sentences usually express action with a strong, clear verb. Compare the verbs in these sentences:

It *is* the committee's recommendation the offer *be given* consideration.

The committee *recommends* that we *consider* the offer.

Recommends and *consider* are more specific than *is* and *be given*. And the verbs in the second version express the important actions of the sentence clearly and directly, rather than burying them in the long *-tion* nouns.

If we regularly express important actions as nouns rather than verbs, our prose will read like the sluggish language so common in business, education, and government.

There is an urgent requirement for an in-depth study of human resource allocation and utilization.

instead of

We must learn how to assign and use our staff more effectively.

Such prose is pompous and inflated. Worse yet, it forces us to wade through it trying to figure out what it means. When a writer relies on excessive nouns and weak verbs, we often find ourselves too fatigued and befuddled to press on. So we reject the document and the message. Check through your writing. If you discover many forms of the verb *to be* (is, was, are, etc.), you may be using too many of the noun forms instead of strong, specific verbs that carry the action of the sentence.

Tell Who Did What

The general rule is simple and often preached by English teachers: Avoid unnecessary passive verbs. The reason: active verbs are usually clearer and less wordy. In addition, active verbs make clear who performed the action of the sentence. *They tell who did what.* The first sentence uses an active verb, the second a passive:

I *closed* the door.

The door *has been closed* by me.

The first sentence is active because the subject performs the action of the sentence. The order is agent–action–goal. Passive constructions reverse that order; the subject does *not* perform the action of the sentence.

Passive constructions have three characteristics:

- The subject does not perform the action of the sentence.
- A form of *to be* always precedes the past participle form of the verb (usually the *-ed* or *-en* form).
- The agent (who or what performs the action) is not stated or is stated in a *by* phrase.

Because of these, overuse of the passive affects your writing in two ways. First, it becomes wordier because of the additional helping verb. This will make your writing bulkier and less energetic. Second, your writing will be more difficult to follow because the passive does not always tell who did what. The reader will therefore have to spend time figuring out precisely what you mean to say.

Those who are fond of passive forms often combine them with deadwood, fancy words, and dull verbs. Here is a passage from a frequently used text on nursing management:

> It is assumed at this point the nurse manager has knowledge of the organizational structures, policies, standards, and job descriptions in force where employment occurs. For purpose of clarity, the concept of direction is divided into two chapters, presenting technologic aspects and interpersonal relationships. . . .It is recognized that in reality, technical activities cannot and should not be separated from human considerations. For this reason there will be some overlap in discussion.

Note the passives: *It is assumed, the concept of direction is divided, It is recognized.* Who assumes, divides, recognizes? Why say *has knowledge of* instead of *knows*? What does *where employment occurs* add to our understanding? We should point out that nurses commit these linguistic crimes no more often than other groups. Such excesses often characterize institutional and academic prose, largely, we think, for the reasons we've cited in our discussion of jargon: habit, to sound important, and so on.

One other reason that the passive so often occurs in business and professional writing is a widespread belief that use of the first-person *I* and *we* is too chatty and informal. If we want to demonstrate our scientific objectivity, we must adopt an aloof third-person style: *it is concluded, therefore, that the experiment can be considered a success* instead of *we conclude that the experiment was a success.* Yet the change in form and the extra words do not change anything. Someone has to be drawing the conclusion, and it is neither nonobjective nor immodest to specify who.

Many writers believe that an impersonal, third-person style is required for publication, in particular. They are convinced that editors won't even consider prose that uses *I* and *we*. This view, however, is incorrect. Look at this paragraph from the conclusion of an article in a recent issue of *Science*, the prestigious publication of the National Association for the Advancement of Science:

> My purpose to this point has been to describe and analyze past events and present trends. Fortune-telling is not my forte, and I do not know what is going to happen after we end our romance with the for-profit health care industry. I do know, however, that we are entering a new era of unprecedented change in the social and economic climate surrounding health care in this country. Academic medicine can influence events by the goals it sets for itself and what it does to achieve those goals.
>
> —Arnold S. Relman, "Who Will Pay for Medical Education in Our Teaching Hospitals?" *Science*, October 5, 1984.

This author, at least, does not believe that the first person is inappropriate to professional communication. And his opinion, we think, counts for a good deal. In addition to being an excellent writer, Dr. Relman is editor of the distinguished *New England Journal of Medicine*. If *I* were a forbidden word in scholarly and scientific articles, he would surely know that and avoid it in his own writing.

Nevertheless, the prejudice against first-person writing is deepseated and persistent. In spite of evidence to the contrary, many of your readers will object that it is too informal and lacks objectivity. So in spite of the fact that you recognize its shortcomings, you may decide that a more formal, "objective" third-person style is sometimes better suited for your audience. In this area of writing as in others, we recommend that you decide what will best serve your goals with particular readers.

Sometimes you may choose to use the passive for other reasons, either because the agent is unimportant (your audience doesn't need to know who's doing it) or because you want to conceal the agent (you don't *want* them to know who's doing it—especially if you did it and it was the wrong thing to do).

The regulation was enacted last year.

Graduate nurses are required to pass an examination before being licensed.

In most circumstances, these sentences would serve better than their active equivalents because no one much cares (or already understands) *who* passed the regulation or requires the examination. Also the subject in both sentences receives the emphasis logically: *the regulation* and *nurses* are what is being talked about in these cases.

One advantage of the active form is that it allows your reader to understand who is the responsible agent. In a sentence such as *The director of nursing has decided that only BSNs will be promoted to management positions,* we understand clearly who has made the decision. A passive version, however, leaves the responsible agent unidentified: *It has been decided that only BSNs will be promoted to management positions.* In most cases, telling the truth and accepting responsibility for one's actions are virtues, in writing as in life. Sometimes, however, you may want to tell less than all the truth, so you might write

This report is being submitted three weeks late.

instead of

I am submitting this report three weeks late.

There are very few inviolable rules in writing, and *avoid the passive in all cases* is not one of them. However, a sensible procedure would be to avoid passive constructions unless you have a specific reason for using one. If you find yourself overusing the passive, try restating your sentences so that they *tell who did what.*

4

Letters
and Résumés

Many of the important documents used by nurses on the job are long and somewhat specialized, and we will discuss them later in this book. But most of the writing you do on the job will be shorter and routine —principally memos and letters. We'll talk about these everyday writing tasks in this chapter and the next. First, however, we'd like to remove some of the mystery from the various sorts of writing you face regularly. If you remember back to Chapter 2, you'll recall that we said that most of the writing you do on the job will have one of two goals or purposes:

- To *inform* your readers of something they need to know, or
- To *persuade* them to do something you want them to do

All of the specialized *forms* of communication you use will be designed to achieve one or both of these goals. Whether you decide to write a letter, memo, or short report is largely irrelevant, provided that the form you choose is appropriate to your subject and audience. In general, however, we can say this about the various forms.

- The *business letter* is generally sent to someone *outside* your institution. In many cases, a letter will be somewhat formal, especially if you do not know the person you're writing to.

- The *memo* is nearly always sent to someone *inside* your institution. It can be formal or informal, depending upon audience and occasion. It is usually short, frequently a single page or less.

- The *informal report* is really nothing more than a longer, more elaborate memo. When used *internally*, it is generally relatively informal, and the distinction between a memo and report may be slight.

- The *formal report*, a longer and more elaborate document than either a memo or informal report, can be used *internally* or *externally*. The formal report usually contains complex information arranged with a number of headings and subheadings.

GENERAL BUSINESS LETTERS

Business writing texts typically divide letters into many categories: inquiry, reply, application, complaint, adjustment, collection, invitation, credit, sales, recommendation, and so on. However, all letters are pretty much alike in that you will always try to produce a document that will be successful with your purpose, topic, and audience. If you use the *SoPA* format we introduced in Chapter 2, a strategy for the letter will probably become clear to you. Obviously, those letters that attempt to persuade a hostile audience will be the most difficult to write, while those that merely communicate information will be easier.

Planning the Letter

Before you begin to write your letter, take a few minutes to think about the two most important elements: your purpose(s) in writing and your reader. Reviewing the *SoPA*, as we have said, will probably help. Make sure you understand precisely what you want to achieve with your letter and how to adapt your purpose to your audience. Make an outline if that helps, or try some of the other ways of getting started that we described at the end of Chapter 2. As you plan your letter, remember that most letters fall logically into a three-part structure: introduction, body, and conclusion.

THE INTRODUCTION

One problem sometimes occurs in the opening of a letter: how do you address it if you don't have the name of someone in particular to write to? Standard practice used to be to use *Gentlemen* as the salutation when writing to a group or organization, perhaps on the assumption that all the members were men (or, perhaps, all the *important* members).Today, for reasons we've discussed in Chapter 3, this no longer serves well. If the recipient is a woman, she might be offended by the implicit assumption that she's male. What to do?

The best solution is to try to find the name of a particular person to address your letter to. A little checking around will sometimes get you the name you need. Failing that, you might try the nonsexist *To Whom It May Concern*. If you seek a fairly formal tone, such a salutation might be appropriate. In some cases, however, it will be too formal and stuffy. An acceptable alternative is *Dear Sir or Madam*, but that, too, is a bit formal (and we're not sure "Madam" is preferable even to "Gentlemen" for some women). We sometimes use the name of the position or organization as a salutation: *Dear Director of Nursing, Dear Bloomingdale's, Dear City Council.* The principal difficulty with any alternative is that it may be either too formal or too informal and therefore put off your reader. In the absence of any clearly agreed-upon practice, we suggest that you first consider the probable effect on your reader. If you don't know or it won't make any difference, use whatever form makes you most comfortable.

Too many letters begin with an opening such as, *I am in receipt of your letter of inquiry dated December 10, 1984.* As someone who understands reader-centered writing, you will quickly recognize one problem with such an opening: it's *writer-centered* rather than *reader-centered.* In addition it wastes too many words. If you're reading a reply letter, you know that the writer has received your letter or he wouldn't be writing back. And you know when you wrote your letter, so you don't need to be reminded. What you want is a quick, clear response, so the writer shouldn't waste words getting to the point.

As the writer of a reply letter, you will occasionally feel compelled to begin with some predictable phrase that constitutes a "proper" opening. Such an opening often comes from habit. And it can offer comfort when you do't know how to begin. But you should resist the temptation to waste words here (or anyplace in your letter). Every paragraph should convey significant information; your first should be a clear, succinct statement of your topic and purpose.

Here are three points to keep in mind for your introduction:

- Get right to your purpose in writing.
- Keep your introduction short.
- See if you can begin with *you* or *thank you*.

This third point is important because it addresses a central psychological fact: the word that most people are more interested in than any other is *you*. If you can begin with this built-in attention grabber, you're well on the way to writing a good reader-centered letter.

As an example, here's the introduction to the "SuperWidget" letter we used in Chapter 1:

Thank you for writing about the SuperWidget Mark II. As the enclosed information indicates, the SuperWidget is comparable in price to other psychomotor regulators but offers you much more.

This short introduction makes clear that the writer is responding to a request for information, that he is enclosing additional information, and that he believes that the SuperWidget offers better value than other regulators.

THE BODY

The introduction introduces your topic; the body develops and explains important details of the topic. To determine how long the body of your letter should be, ask yourself how many important points your reader needs to know in order to understand and if necessary act on your topic. Here, for example, is the three-paragraph body of the "SuperWidget" letter:

Its recycling time is .05 seconds, considerably faster than the usual .20 seconds of similar equipment. This means faster turnaround time with patients and more effective use of valuable nurses' time.

In addition, the new technology in the SuperWidget makes it extremely accurate and reliable. We have recently installed units at Sagamon Valley Hospital and Lakeview Community Hospital. I hope you will contact your colleagues about their reaction to the SuperWidget.

Printed materials alone cannot reveal all the features of the SuperWidget, so I have asked Walter Johnson, our upstate New York representative, to contact you for an appointment. Mr. Johnson will be happy to demonstrate the SuperWidget to you and your staff.

Each paragraph of the body makes a separate, detailed point: (1) that the SuperWidget is faster and more effective than competitors; (2) that it is accurate and reliable according to nurses in nearby hospitals; (3) that the writer has arranged for a demonstration of the machine in the recipient's hospital.

In the body of your letter, your paragraphs may be longer than in your introduction or conclusion. Remember that each paragraph should discuss one logical unit—a single point or a group of closely related points. Furthermore, the sentences within each paragraph should be arranged in some logical (or psychological) order—the order that does the most to support your purpose. You will usually want to place the more important details at the beginning or end of your paragraphs, the less important details in the middle, which receives less emphasis.

Effective paragraphs reflect not only a sensible order of details but also coherence. Paragraphs cohere (from the Latin, "stick together") if you provide effective signals to the reader so that she knows how the ideas you include relate to one another. You can help create coherence through effective transitions that guide your reader from one idea to another, one sentence to another. In particular, two types of words and phrases can help your reader understand the relationships between ideas in your paragraphs.

Pronouns.   Whenever you use a pronoun, the reader will unconsciously recall the antecedent (the noun the pronoun refers back to) of the word you use. In the first paragraph of the three shown above, two pronouns work in this way. *Its* refers back to the SuperWidget mentioned in the introductory paragraph and thus shows the connection of the introductory paragraph to what follows. And *this* in the second sentence refers back to the quick recycling time. Each time you use a pronoun in this way, you help create links between your ideas, making them clearer and easier for the reader to follow.

Transitional Words and Phrases.   Transitional words and phrases create an explicit link between sentences and ideas, showing that two things are related and, in some cases, specifying the nature of the relationship. In the lists below, you will find some of the more common and useful.

Transitions to show time: later, next, first, second, third, before, after, suddenly, now, then, in the past, in the future, thereafter, previously, afterwards, often

Transitions to show place or location: there, above, below, against, on, beside, around, beyond, forward, backward, in front of, alongside, inside, outside, through

Transitions to show logical relationships:

> *Addition and comparison:*   in addition, likewise, and, moreover, besides, again, too, furthermore, further, next, last, also, similarly, likewise

> *Contrast or differences:*   but, still, however, nonetheless, nevertheless, on the contrary, after all, even though, though, on the other hand, in contrast, yet, in spite of

> *Result or consequence:*   thus, as a result, consequently, accordingly, therefore, because, since, hence, for

> *Summary:*   therefore, finally, as a result, all in all, accordingly, in other words, in summary, in conclusion

> *Emphasis:*   surely, certainly, to be sure, indeed, in fact, truly, without a doubt, undoubtedly

> *Indicating that an example will follow:*   for example, as an example, for instance, to illustrate, as proof, as an illustration

> *To qualify or restrict an idea:*   if, provided, when, in the case of, unless, frequently, occasionally, in particular, in general, specifically, especially, usually

Using Lists.   One problem can occur when you need to make a large number of points within a single paragraph or letter. How can you present them so as to keep the information as clear as possible to the reader? One effective solution that is little used by business writers is a simple *list*. Lists have two virtues: they are clear and easy to follow, and they emphasize the material they contain. You will notice that we have used them throughout this book for both reasons. You should not hesitate to use them in your writing.

Here is a short checklist of points to keep in mind for the body of your letter:

- Use each paragraph to explain a single point or group of closely related points.
- Determine a sensible order for your points.
- Use transitional words and phrases to achieve coherence.
- Consider lists to clarify when appropriate.

THE CONCLUSION

Many writers commit the same error in concluding their letters that they do in introducing them: employing lifeless, predictable language that serves virtually no purpose. Every sentence in your letter should say something; so avoid formula conclusions. Instead, concentrate on making use of the conclusion to help achieve your purpose in writing the letter. If your letter is long or particularly complex, you may need to summarize main points, but don't do that unless it's necessary. If your letter contains welcome news, you may want to reiterate it. Any time you can close your letter on a positive note, it's good to do it. Your conclusion is particularly important in establishing the tone of your letter because it is the last thing the reader reads.

As a conclusion to our discussion of conclusions, we suggest that you keep these points in mind:

- Avoid overused "formula" phrases.
- If necessary, summarize your main points.
- Try to conclude on a positive note.

Letter Formats

We don't think that a detailed discussion of all the subtleties (some would say perversities) of letter format is very important or useful. Most business letters are typed by someone other than the writer, so worrying about spacing, paragraphing, arrangement, and other such matters is ridiculous. No one format is universally prescribed. Several can be correct, and unless yours is clearly odd, no one will be likely to notice it. If you have a secretary, rely on him or her to come up with the correct details. Most secretarial courses and manuals teach the arcane matters of letter form. If you do not have a secretary, follow the format used by your institution or by the person writing to you. If you can't even find a sample letter to follow, most English handbooks, some dictionaries, and all secretarial manuals will help you through the details. Given a choice between various formats, choose the one that looks best to you. Two general styles are common: block and modified block.

BLOCK FORMAT

In *block* format, every line begins at the left margin, so the typist has to make very few adjustments before beginning to type and while typing. Many businesses have adopted this form because it saves busy secretaries time. It is very simple but has a singular disadvantage: because everything is lined up on the left margin, the letter generally looks like it's tilting to the port side. Figure 4.1 gives an example: our SuperWidget letter written in strict block format.

MODIFIED BLOCK FORMAT

We think the few seconds saved in typing the letter does not make up for the fact that this format is often unpleasing to the eye. So we prefer *modified block* format (as do about ¾ of business letter writers). This style is similar to the block format, but the date, the complimentary close, name of the writer, and title are usually placed at (or five spaces to the right of) the center line of the paper. Figure 4.2 shows the same letter written in modified block format.

W I D G E T C O R P , I N C
2880 National Highway
Quahog, NY 14855

January 25, 1985

Ms. Donna Wilson, R.N.
Head Nurse, Psychiatric Unit
Happy Valley Hospital
Port Cayuga, NY 14851

Dear Ms. Wilson:

Thank you for writing about the SuperWidget Mark II. As the enclosed information indicates, the SuperWidget is comparable in price to other psychomotor regulators but offers you much more.

Its recycling time is .05 seconds, considerably faster than the usual .20 seconds of similar equipment. This means faster turnaround time with patients and more effective use of valuable nurses' time.

In addition, the new technology in the SuperWidget makes it extremely accurate and reliable. We have recently installed units at Sagamon Valley Hospital and Lakeview Community Hospital. I hope you will contact your colleagues about their reaction to the SuperWidget.

Printed materials alone cannot reveal all the features of the SuperWidget, so I have asked Walter Johnson, our upstate New York representative, to contact you for an appointment. Mr. Johnson will be happy to demonstrate the SuperWidget to you and your staff.

Once you see the SuperWidget in operation, I am sure you will agree that it offers the best combination of features available today. Thank you for your interest in SuperWidget.

Sincerely,

E.B. Sahl
National Sales Manager

EBS:eb

Enclosure

Figure 4.1. A letter typed in block form. Note that all lines start on the left margin.

W I D G E T C O R P , I N C
2880 National Highway
Quahog, NY 14855

January 25, 1985

Ms. Donna Wilson, R.N.
Head Nurse, Psychiatric Unit
Happy Valley Hospital
Port Cayuga, NY 14851

Dear Ms. Wilson:

Thank you for writing about the SuperWidget Mark II. As the enclosed information indicates, the SuperWidget is comparable in price to other psychomotor regulators but offers you much more.

Its recycling time is .05 seconds, considerably faster than the usual .20 seconds of similar equipment. This means faster turnaround time with patients and more effective use of valuable nurses' time.

In addition, the new technology in the SuperWidget makes it extremely accurate and reliable. We have recently installed units at Sagamon Valley Hospital and Lakeview Community Hospital. I hope you will contact your colleagues about their reaction to the SuperWidget.

Printed materials alone cannot reveal all the features of the SuperWidget, so I have asked Walter Johnson, our upstate New York representative, to contact you for an appointment. Mr. Johnson will be happy to demonstrate the SuperWidget to you and your staff.

Once you see the SuperWidget in operation, I am sure you will agree that it offers the best combination of features available today. Thank you for your interest in SuperWidget.

Sincerely,

E.B. Sahl
National Sales Manager

EBS:eb

Enclosure

Figure 4.2. A letter typed in modified block form. Note that date and closing lines are slightly to the right of the center of the page.

These formats are shown on letterhead, but would not be essentially different if you were using plain paper. In that case, you would simply type your own address directly above the date at the top of the page. The whole thing is not nearly as mysterious as it is often made out to be. Simply pay attention to the way the letter looks on the page and arrange things so that the finished letter looks nice to you.

Problem Letters: Saying What Your Reader Doesn't Want to Hear

Some letters are particularly difficult to write because you must convey unpleasant information to your reader. Presenting bad news effectively is an art that we all can benefit from thinking more about. By the time you have completed your analysis of purpose and reader, you will have an idea of how to go about approaching the reader who isn't going to like what you have to say. In addition to the obvious points, such as trying to understand how your reader will feel about what you have to say, we'd like to offer three suggestions about conveying bad news:

- Be courteous.
- Be positive.
- Slip the bad news in gently.

BE COURTEOUS

Courtesy is so obviously important in writing business letters (as it is in most human endeavors) that it almost seems unnecessary to mention it. But it's useful to all of us to be reminded of how important it is, even when we have only a few minutes to compose a letter. You're not likely to be deliberately discourteous except when angry. That's a very good reason for not writing when you *are* angry. (We know a former university administrator who used to compose his fiery letters, then let them sit in his desk overnight. The next morning he would reread them and throw them away. That way, he received the satisfaction of skewering someone but didn't suffer the consequences of actually sending the inappropriately phrased letter.)

Even when we're not angry, we may inadvertently be tactless or insulting to a reader because we fail to realize how a reader will react to our words or tone. Consider these examples, with the offending phrases italicized:

> Because *you failed* to include a detailed budget, we cannot award you the contract.
>
> *You should know* that a ten-year-old toaster will not be covered by warranty.

With a bit more concern for the feelings of readers, these sentences could have been rewritten to avoid giving offense:

> Because a detailed budget was not included, we cannot award you the contract.
>
> Since you have owned your toaster for ten years, it is no longer covered by warranty.

BE POSITIVE

Our second piece of advice, *be positive*, is sometimes more difficult to follow. If you are writing a letter to fire someone, for example, you may not be able to think of anything other than the negatives that led to the dismissal. But with some thought you will often be able to say precisely the same thing in positive rather than negative terms. Consider these pairs of sentences:

> Central supply closes at 6:45 p.m.
> Central supply is open until 6:45 p.m.

> We can't consider your application until we receive three letters of recommendation.
> We will be able to consider your application as soon as we receive three letters of recommendation.

The same point is highlighted in a writing experiment we've heard described. A group of students were assigned to compose letters of refusal to a woman who had experienced a problem with some jars for home canning. She reported that the lids had failed to seat properly, and she requested to be reimbursed for her destroyed fruit, the lids, and her labor. She mentioned in her request that all of the three dozen lids she purchased had failed. The students were informed that company quality control tests showed that only about one per cent of the lids failed when used with reasonable care. The students used this information to support their contention that the lids were probably not the cause of the problem. Nearly all the students, however, phrased the test results in negative terms: *only one per cent of the lids failed to seal.* Just one emphasized the positive: *99 per cent of the lids sealed perfectly.*

Choosing the positive word is often merely a matter of perspective and emphasis. The principle is the same as the one illustrated by the story of the glass of water: is it half empty or half full? It's the same glass and the same water, but it can be described negatively or positively, depending upon how you look at the situation. Your attitude toward any issue can influence the tone of your letter. Does that staff nurse *seldom make mistakes* or is she *nearly always correct?* The performance of the new ward clerk might be described as *not bad.* How is that different from *generally good?* If you choose the positive, your words will influence the whole tone of your letter, making it more appealing (and so more effective) to the reader.

SLIP THE BAD NEWS IN GENTLY

Finally, we suggest that you deliver the bad news delicately. By that we don't mean that you should adopt rosy euphemisms and say that the patient "passed on" instead of "died." In a sense, we're describing a variety of the point we've just mentioned: just as you should emphasize the positive, it's useful sometimes to de-emphasize the negative. Here's an example that comes from our own university.

Dear Mike,

As you requested, I'm sending word of your final grade before I leave town for the holidays. Your work in the beginning of the semester was quite good, in particular your fine paper on Fitzgerald's *The Great Gatsby.*

However, your last paper and your final exam were not up to that standard. Although you said some good things in your paper on Housman's "To An Athlete Dying Young," you overlooked the important point that dying young and in glory might be preferable to living so long that "the name died before the man." With the C+ on that paper and a disappointing C on the final exam, I'm afraid that your average works out to less than the B you had hoped to receive. I've had to turn in a C as your final grade. It was a high C, however, and I believe that you'll do better in the future, especially as you become more accustomed to living away from home and learn to budget your time more effectively.

I enjoyed having you as a student, especially your lively sense of humor and willingness to speak up in class. I hope we'll meet again, either in another of my classes or by your dropping by my office occasionally.

Sincerely,

John Clare

This letter, we think, incorporates all the guidelines we've been suggesting. It manages to be courteous, as positive as possible, and sensitive to the reader's feelings. Although it reports the fact that Mike received a C for the course, that negative is de-emphasized and softened by the explanation that precedes it and the encouragement that follows. To see why this is effective, put yourself in Mike's position and imagine precisely the same letter beginning with this sentence: *I'm sorry to have to tell you that your grade for the course is a C.* In the sample letter, Mike already knows what the bad news will be before he gets there. Because the letter offers the reasons first and then the decision, he will have a chance to assimilate them. Many people would simply tune out the remainder of the letter if it began with the "I'm sorry to have to say" sentence. So placing the bad news in the middle of the letter and building toward it with reasons offered beforehand accomplishes two things. It ensures that Mike will understand *why* he earned the C, and it will prepare him in advance for the news he doesn't want to hear.

APPLICATION LETTERS

Most people write only a few application letters in a whole career, but those few are very important, for the end result is success or failure in getting a job. Both make the application letter difficult to write: so much depends upon it, and you write one so seldom. Therefore, we'll look at some of the special qualities of the letter of application and (in the next section) the résumé.

Understand Your Audience

In some ways, the job application letter is no different than any other persuasive document. It is essentially a sales letter; you're selling yourself—your training, experience, abilities, and character. Often you will be responding to an advertisement, so you know you will have an interested reader, someone who wants to hire the best person for the job. Your principal goal is not to get the job, however, it is to *get the interview*. Therefore you want to design a letter-and-résumé package that is sufficiently interesting to persuade the hirer to call you for an interview.

Your task calls for a particularly careful audience analysis: *precisely* what is the hirer likely to be looking for in an applicant? How can you match your own qualifications to what you understand to be the needs of the employer? First of all, you may need to do some homework. What do you know—or what can you find out—about the institution? Is it identified with a particular mission, specialty, or religious group? Does it have a particularly strong reputation or does it need strengthening in some area? What is its management philosophy? The more you can learn about the place, the better you can tailor your letter to that particular audience.

Present Yourself Effectively

For most of you reading this book, an application letter will not be your first: perhaps you're ready to move into management or to take another step higher on your career ladder. That means you have accumulated some good experience and developed skills since you left training. Take a moment to assess your qualifications. What are your strengths as a potential or actual manager? Remember that employers may be more interested in your managerial skills than your nursing, at least at the level above head nurse. You will need to think about how you can demonstrate your abilities to communicate, motivate, analyze, solve problems, and organize. Decide how you can best present yourself to the employer who needs you but doesn't yet *know* that.

Remember to use the letter and résumé together. Make sure that every important aspect of your qualifications is included in one or the other; emphasize particularly strong points by including them in both. You may have been told that both letter and résumé should be no more than one page long. Nonsense. Though that may be true for people seeking their first job, by now you have accumulated a substantial record of knowledge and experience. Don't slight your strengths by arbitrarily compressing them onto a single page. It is true that *all things being equal* shorter is better. Employers may not have the time or the inclination to wade through bulky materials, and documents that are obviously padded won't be taken seriously. Also, you must consider personal preferences of your readers if you know them. We know of one personnel person who simply will not read an application letter longer than one page. But we have heard about him precisely because such behavior is unusual. If you know you're writing to him you'll certainly want to keep your letter short. But the general principle to keep in mind is this: the employer wants to hire the best person for the job. The more she or he knows about how well you meet the qualifications, the better for both of you.

As former administrators, we've formed our own opinions about appropriate lengths for letters and résumés. In general, we prefer to see letters of about one page, and never longer than two. Résumés can vary from just a page or two for people early in their careers to five pages or even longer in the case of experienced, accomplished professionals. (As an example, ours are four and five pages, respectively, including publications.) Be succinct and don't pad, but be sure to include all relevant information.

Organize Your Letter Effectively

The parts of an application letter correspond to the parts of general business letters we've identified above, but they serve special functions as you tailor your letter to the job and your qualifications.

INTRODUCTION

The first paragraph will usually involve only a sentence or two. If you can mention a name or two that might help your cause, do it. If you're responding to an advertisement, refer to it. Be specific about the position you're applying for: the institution may have more than one open at a time. If you can write to a specific individual, that's best. Even if no name is mentioned in the ad, see if you can find out the name of the director of nursing or some other appropriate person; your effort will probably be noticed.

The introduction need not be jazzy or inflated, but you should begin as strongly as possible. One strategy is to associate one of your strengths with one of the requirements for the job. Try to get as much valuable information to the employer as early as possible. Don't settle for pat, standard openings like these:

> Enclosed please find a brief résumé of my training and experience in nursing management.
>
> I am writing this letter with reference to your advertisement in the *AJN*.

These are wasted words: they do little to advance your case and because they're dull and lifeless don't encourage anyone to read beyond the first sentence.

Compare these openings that really say something:

> Florence Styxx, my Director of Nursing, has suggested that I write to you about the evening supervisor position you are seeking to fill. Because I have held a number of management positions and am now head nurse on a large medical unit, she believes you may be interested in my application.
>
> My family and I will be moving to the Philadelphia area soon, so I was particularly interested to read your advertisement for a Director of Nursing in today's *Inquirer*. As a master's prepared nurse with extensive experience as a clinical specialist and supervisor in a large general hospital and a regional children's hospital, I believe I can offer the qualifications you seek.

Both of these openings lead with strengths. In the first example, the writer assumes that the fact that his current director suggested that he apply will have a positive effect. The opening implies that the writer has proved himself as a head nurse and is now ready to move up. Presumably, Florence Styxx thinks highly of his performance and will provide a reference if asked.

The second example is somewhat different. Because she is from a different city, the writer states that she will be moving to Philadelphia, then goes on to mention what she considers to be her strengths: her master's degree and administrative experience in two different kinds of hospital. In both cases, the writers have indicated what positions they are applying for and how they learned about them, but have also combined that information with reasons why they should be considered for the jobs—all this in just two sentences.

BODY

In the body of your letter, you will want to expand upon the information contained in your résumé (but don't just repeat it). Explain why your background matches the employer's requirements. Emphasize your strengths. Explain any apparent weaknesses or shortcomings in your résumé. The 18 months you worked at Barb's Burger Bar when you lived in a small town just after you got married might be a problem. But if you explain that there were no nursing vacancies in the local 30-bed hospital and that you gained valuable supervisory experience at B. B. B., that could be a strength rather than a weakness.

Try to anticipate any questions that the employer might have. If you didn't work for two years, explain why. Taking time to raise a child or help your wife with her business is legitimate; two years in prison isn't. How will the employer know if you don't mention the reason for the hiatus?

Pay particular attention to the strengths in your qualifications, and explain them as fully as necessary. If you had a graduate course with a well-known professor, took part in a clinical research study, helped rewrite the policy and procedure manuals, received an award for streamlining a hospital procedure, or had an article published, describe your experience in as much detail as is required for the employer to understad how it relates to the position you seek. Don't boast, but don't be overly modest either. If you don't blow your own horn (however discreetly), no one else is likely to blow it for you.

Be honest, direct, and positive (but not overbearing). The employer wants to hire the right *person*, not just a set of qualifications, so you want to communicate an accurate sense of your individuality as well as your training and experience. Try to sustain a tone that is appropriate to the employer and you. Make your letter reader-centered, and try not to overuse the word *I*. You can't avoid using a few *I*'s but don't make your letter one of those that overwhelms the reader with them: it will make you sound appallingly self-centered.

CONCLUSION

Request something specific from the reader. Indicate you are available for an interview, can come to her office, or will be in town on a certain date. Specify where and when you can be reached. If appropriate, reiterate a significant point you made earlier in the letter, reminding the reader yet again of one of your principal strengths. Here are two examples:

> Because my experience seems to be a good match with the qualifications you have stated, I would like very much to speak with you in person about the position. I will be in Philadelphia from May 11–15 and may be reached at the home of my sister, Kate Benjamin, 216-488-3850. I look forward to meeting you.

> After you have examined the attached résumé, please call or write and suggest a time when we can meet to discuss the position and my qualifications in more detail. I work steady days, so late afternoon would be the most convenient time for an interview, but I would be happy to arrange another time if you would like.

Some Special Considerations

Writing the letter of application sometimes involves problems not usually encountered in other types of letters. They can be difficult and require special care if you encounter them.

The Question of Salary.   Some advertisements will ask you to state the salary you expect, though most do not. This poses a difficult problem: do I risk not getting the job if my figure is too high, or getting less than I'm worth if it's too low? The answer is "probably not" in both cases. Most positions are budgeted at a fairly specific range, though positions with higher salaries and more responsibility may have a good deal of negotiating flexibility. If you have a minimum salary beneath which you would not accept a job, by all means state it. If it's close to what the employer has in mind, he can sometimes be flexible. If not, we prefer to try to sidestep the issue. You can do this in various ways:

> I would expect a salary appropriate to my qualifications and the responsibilities of the position.

> Although salary is less important than the challenges and satisfactions of the position, I would expect to receive something in the range of $25,000–30,000.

> My current salary is $29,800 per year. It would be very difficult for me to consider a position that did not at least equal that.

However, we recommend that you never bring up the matter of money unless it's critically important to you. If the employer becomes interested in you, there will be time enough to discuss salary later. You should, however, be prepared to answer questions about expected salary if you progress to the interview stage. If you want to be as flexible as possible, consider some variation on the phrasing above for use when you're asked.

Confidentiality. If you don't want your employer to know you're looking for another job, be sure to indicate that in your letter. Some people routinely check with an applicant's supervisor before deciding whom to interview. However, a prospective employer who is interested in you will almost always delay speaking to your current employer if you ask. (But do not assume that your employer will *never* be contacted). A sentence like this will usually solve the problem:

> Please do not contact my present employer until we have established a mutual interest in pursuing discussions about the position.

Many employers have been in similar positions themselves, and such a request will usually be honored.

Summary

Keep these points in mind when you write your application letter.

- Gather the information necessary to make your letter reader-centered.
- Write a strong, relevant introduction.

- Supply supporting details in the body.
- Make the tone of your letter confident but not pushy.
- Make your letter amplify and explain your résumé, not just repeat it.
- Write a strong, positive conclusion.

RÉSUMÉS

Like letters, résumés have generated a good deal of mystery for no good reason. (A résumé is also known as a *curriculum vitae,* or *vita* for short, principally in academic circles. For all practical purposes, a résumé and a *vita* are identical.) The purpose of a résumé is quite simple: to present a prospective employer with enough information about you to lead to an interview. Remember that your résumé will be paired with your letter of application and that the two should work together. If your application letter is short, your résumé should be more detailed (or vice versa). The letter should include some points from the résumé and explain or expand upon them. The résumé should contain all the important information about you that is necessary for the employer to decide that you're a good prospect for the job. As we've said above, the résumé (like the application letter) should be long enough to include *all* important information without being padded.

The Function of a Résumé

Many people think that a résumé is merely a data sheet, but that's a mistake. If all you include is bare facts, you might as well just fill out the institution's application form (which you'll probably have to do anyway) and forget it. It's not true that "the facts speak for themselves," for most facts need to be interpreted. That, basically, is a central function of your résumé—not just to list the facts of your education, experience, and so on, but to *arrange* and *interpret* them.

Don't Follow Someone Else's Form

No doubt you have prepared a résumé at some point. Many people we know keep one up-to-date and handy. But we have seen very few really effective résumés. One reason is that most people seem to have followed some sort of form, perhaps one they were given as they sought their first job after school, but without any clear thought about whether that form is effective for their individual characteristics.

Because you're a unique individual, you have unique characteristics to offer an employer. No single form can allow for your individuality, so it's a mistake to follow one slavishly. You should *build your résumé around your strengths.* Make it fit you rather than trying to fit someone else's arrangement. Of course there are a number of elements that employers will expect to see on the résumé: job experience, education, personal characteristics, perhaps references and a job objective statement. But it is up to you how and where to include them. Seek an arrangement that emphasizes your strong points, minimizes your weaknesses.

For example, most résumés routinely list education before experience. That might be the best arrangement for someone just out of school, someone whose work experience is limited. (One reason for this being such a common form is that many sample résumés are prepared by placement offices or other services designed to help graduates get their first professional jobs.) When experience is more relevant and stronger than training, however, it's foolish to lead with the weaker category. Start right off with what you want to emphasize. For most experienced professionals, education was just a starting point in the more or less distant past. The skills and knowledge gained more recently will be more important. But if you recently completed a graduate program, for example, you may want to highlight that fact.

What to Include

Most résumés will have all or most of these categories of information, but not necessarily precisely these headings or this arrangement:

Heading: Including name, address, telephone number.

Personal data: In recent years, there has been a trend away from including much personal data, resulting partly from antidiscrimination legislation. Consequently, you're not obliged to include much if any. But you may *want* to include information that you believe will increase your prospects for landing the job.

Employment objective: If you have a specific job in mind, list it; if not, you could list two or three possibilities, a general statement, or leave this element out.

Licensure: List your licenses, with state, number, and date.

Professional specialization: You may want to indicate one or two areas of clinical specialization, either here or under your employment objective or employment experience sections.

Employment experience: Usually begin with the most recent and provide dates of employment, name and address of employer, job title, and a brief description of duties and responsibilities. You may also want to include any special qualifications or outstanding achievements on the job. Service in the armed forces would also be included here.

Education: Begin with the most recent and work backwards. Provide dates attended, degree or certificate earned, and information on courses related to your employment objective. Once again, highlight your strengths. Be sure to include any scholarships or honors, your grade average (if it was high), and other details that set you apart from the average student.

Supporting data: If you have acquired any special skills but are not sure where to put them, you might group them together or create a special category: languages, membership in professional societies, publications, workshops presented, job-related hobbies. Unless they are extensive, you may want to try to include these details under education and experience.

References: You may either list your references (after checking with them, of course) or say: *References provided upon request.* Decide which would be better for you. If one of your references is well-known, you might want to include names. But perhaps you're selecting different references for different positions, in which case you won't want to list them. Unless you have a specific reason for not wanting to do so, however, we think it's best to list your references (with addresses and telephone numbers so that they can be contacted quickly and easily).

Design an Attractive Format

There are so many possible formats for your résumé that we've resisted giving you one or two samples. Even our own are strikingly different in arrangement and emphasis, and we want you to practice what we've been preaching: *design your own format to present your own qualifications effectively.* We do, however, offer two additional suggestions:

- Give careful consideration to how you arrange your résumé on the page. The importance of appearance cannot be overemphasized. An attractive résumé will draw favorable attention to you. One that is cramped or badly arranged will work against you.

- Make absolutely sure that your résumé and your application letter are completely free of errors. Even one small mistake can damage the favorable impression you hope to make. Proofread your letter and résumé carefully before you send them out. Ask someone else to check them over for you as well.

By following the guidelines we've offered in this chapter, you will be able to create letters and résumés that present you in the best possible light and increase your chances of achieving your purposes in writing.

5

Memos
and Reports

"I love being a manager, but I hate to write all these memos and reports. Why can't I spend my time more constructively?" We have found this is a common sentiment among nurse managers. It develops, we think, because of the frustration associated with putting pen to paper, not because you believe that reporting information is necessarily a waste of time. In fact, reporting has always been an integral part of nursing practice. What would happen to patient care if we did not report to other nurses, physicians, or patients? Granted, the types of reports required of a manager are more complex than those directly associated with patient care. And it's often the indirect association with patient care that leads to some of the frustration with writing memos and reports.

This chapter will focus on several different forms for reporting information: memos, informal reports, and formal reports. We'll examine various formats and kinds of reports and present a sample of a long formal report using statistical information in various forms. While this chapter will not cover every possible type of report that you might be asked to write, it will give you most of what you need to prepare any document you're likely to be called on to write.

GENERAL POINTS TO CONSIDER

Memos and reports are used principally for *internal* communications, when you need to inform, instruct, or persuade someone within your organization. Rather than being clearly distinct forms, memos and reports form a continuum of length and complexity. At one end would be a very short memo, at the other an elaborate, full-blown formal report complete with many headings and subheadings. The memo is usually informal in tone (though not always), while a long report is nearly always much more formal in both tone and structure. In essence, then, we're talking about three kinds of reports: memo reports, informal reports, and formal reports. Broadly defined, almost any communication of facts, ideas, or opinions is a report.

What is important, of course, is not defining a report but writing it. If you examine reports written in your institution, you will probably recognize some common shortcomings. These include poor organization of ideas, lack of consideration of the audience, flabby language, inconsistency in tone and style, lack of clarity, and unclear directions. We've described how to avoid most of these pitfalls in Chapters 1, 2, and 3.

When you have to write a report, the most important question you should ask yourself is "What is the purpose of this document?" The SoPA form we presented in Chapter 2 offers a helpful way to address this question. If you don't clearly understand why you are writing the document, your reader almost certainly won't get much from it. For example, suppose you are asked to report on overtime in your department. Where do you begin? Does your boss expect a short summary of overtime hours worked or a complete analysis of the causes and effects of the overtime? Should you report on overtime for last week, last month, or last year?

At this point, you need to find out exactly what your boss expects. You should do that with a phone call, a chat in the hall, or—more formally—a short memo in which you describe various approaches to the report and determine which is most appropriate. You may not want to bother the boss or reveal your ignorance of what she expects. But aren't you better off doing that than writing a report that does not provide what she wanted?

Once you've determined your specific task, you can think about which format would be the most appropriate: memo, informal report, or formal report.

MEMOS

Memo, of course, is short for *memorandum*, perhaps the most frequently used form of communication in any institution. Unlike letters, memos are used almost exclusively to communicate to people within the agency or institution. Most institutions provide their own forms, usually with spaces for:

DATE:
TO:
FROM:
SUBJECT:

Some printed forms may be arranged differently, but this is the basic information that should appear at the head of your memos. Don't neglect the *Subject* line (sometimes abbreviated as *Subj* or *Re)*, even if it's not on your agency's form, for it performs an important function in all but the shortest memos. Think of it as being equivalent to the title of a report or a newspaper headline. It alerts the reader to the subject of the memo, so your topic is clear before the reader gets to the text itself. She can devote all her attention to your message without having to figure what you're writing about.

Memos serve many purposes, among them:

- Giving information or direction
- Defining a problem
- Providing procedures or instructions
- Explaining or justifying your actions

All of these could just as easily be the topics for informal reports, too. As we've said, the difference between a memo and a report is principally a matter of length and complexity. If your topic can be dealt with in just a page or two, you'll probably write a memo. If it requires more discussion because it's more complex or needs more documentation, you'll produce an informal report. One shades into the other. Distinctions between them are not very important.

Like a business letter, a memo is divided functionally into three parts:

- *Introduction:* states the purpose of the memo and summarizes its most important points.
- *Body* or *discussion:* explains the most important points, or offers evidence or reasons.
- *Conclusion:* tells the reader what to think about, what to do, what to expect next.

But a memo will frequently be much shorter than a letter; all three of the functional parts could conceivably be included in three sentences, or even one:

I will be away from the office for two weeks beginning August 1. In my absence, Elizabeth Garver will be acting as evening supervisor. Please direct your problems or questions to her while I am away.

While I am away from the hospital, Elizabeth Garver will be acting supervisor and will answer your questions until I return.

You should of course remember to make your memo as clear as possible, reader-centered, and to-the-point. Unfortunately, not all writers achieve these goals, and the memo is therefore the most abused as well as the most used form of communication. Here is an actual example brought in to one of our classes, reproduced exactly (but with names changed to protect the guilty):

MEMORANDUM
ST. ELIJAH'S MEDICAL CENTER

Date: May 7, 1984

To: Mr. James Schmidt, Laundry Manager

From: Sr. Suzanne Kolter, Assistant Director, Housekeeping

Re: "Caron" Pillow With Blue Cover

These pillows <u>do not</u> get washed by laundry department, <u>do not</u> put a pillow cover on pillow just a pillow case.

If something is spilled on them during the patient stay <u>Nursing Service should just wipe it off at the time.</u>

<u>Upon discharge,</u> the <u>discharge unit service</u> will wash the pillow just like the mattress.

In many ways, this memo is so bad as to be funny. It is filled with sentence errors and sprinkled with unnecessary underlining for emphasis. But even those errors, irritating though they may be, are insignificant in comparison to the memo's confusion and lack of awareness of audience. What does the writer want to say and to whom? The memo is addressed to the laundry but speaks also of the responsibilities of two other units. Why is the writer telling the laundry what "Nursing Services" and "the discharge unit service" should do, especially since there's no indication that she's sending the same information to those units?

If you were the recipient, how would you react to this memo? Although we find it unintentionally hilarious, the recipient probably didn't. He was probably confused and angry at being addressed in such a fashion. The writer has committed at least three serious errors:

- The memo is filled with errors.
- It doesn't make clear its purpose (why was it written?).
- Its tone is offensive.

Here's a much more effective memo (with the names once again changed):

SHENANGO VALLEY COMMUNITY HOSPITAL
MEMORANDUM

To:	John Valdez, Clinical Specialist	Date:	November 17, 1984
From:	Betty Pankowsky, Home Health Agency	Subj:	Follow-up Treatment for Tim Johnson

I have just learned from Dr. Swanson that Mr. Johnson is recovering well from his amputation and that he will be discharged early next week. He has been assigned to me for home health care, and I would like to ask you about these matters:

1. Is he experiencing any difficulties with his prosthesis?
2. How is he adapting emotionally?
3. Are there special factors I should know about?

In addition, I would appreciate any suggestions you can make concerning follow-up therapy for Mr. Johnson. Thank you very much.

This memo is admirable in a number of ways. It's reader-centered and reveals a good sense of audience. Because it's succinct and well-organized, it is easily understood by the reader. Finally, it makes clear what it wants from the reader. It serves its purpose well.

INFORMAL REPORTS

In short reports, the organization is not as formalized or complicated as in long reports. Provided that your report is no more than a few pages (say three or four), you need not worry about such matters as a title page, table of contents, abstract, and so on. But remember that the function of any document's form is to help the reader understand what you want to communicate. The organization you choose should clearly indicate what you're doing and where you're going in the report.

The informal report is divided functionally into the now-familiar three parts: introduction, body (discussion), and conclusion. These sections may or may not have separate headings. Decide whether they are necessary based upon the length and complexity of your document. For example, a two-page report recommending some changes in scheduling might be presented in memo form with the following heading and introduction:

MEMORANDUM

Date: December 29, 1984

From: Annette Williamson, Patient Care Coordinator

To: Stacy Amato, Director of Nursing Services

Subj: Recommendations for Changes in Scheduling Staff Nurses

The purpose of this report is to recommend changes in our methods of scheduling staff nurses. The discussion first summarizes our present procedures, then identifies some of the problems, and concludes with recommendations to correct the problems.

This introduction makes clear how the report is organized, so separate internal headings are probably unnecessary. However, if the report were longer or the material complex, the writer might well want to present it in a different form: a short report with internal headings accompanied by a cover memo. In that case, the example we've shown above might serve as the separate cover memo, and the report itself might have the following headings to reflect the organization:

Current Scheduling Procedures

Problems with the Current System

Recommendations

Depending upon length and complexity, your informal report might include any of the possible parts of an extended formal report:

Preliminary Material

   Cover page

   Foreword

   Title page

   Contents page

   Summary or abstract

Introduction

Body (Discussion)

   Purpose

   Methods or procedures

   Findings

Conclusion and/or Recommendations

Addenda

   Bibliography or References

   Appendix

   Index

Not even fully developed formal reports will necessarily contain all these parts, but any report may contain some of them. Shorter reports will be less formal and contain fewer. In a short memo report, you may not need to display any subheadings. Longer reports will require more of the parts and more labels to help guide the reader through them. The central point to remember, though, is that only you can decide what format is appropriate for your purpose, your subject, and your audience. If a short, simple report will be adequate, use it. That will be easier for you and your reader. But if your subject or audience demands a long, elaborate, formal report, use it.

FORMAL REPORTS

The degree of a report's formality usually depends on its intended audience and the use(s) to which it will be put. Is it for readers inside or outside the institution, department, or division? Is the topic well understood or not? Will the reader expect a particular tone or length? Another important factor is the length and complexity of analysis undertaken in the report. Complex, lengthy analyses may require more supporting detail and a more elaborate structure than simpler matters. In the following pages, we'll discuss some of the special kinds of reports that nurse managers frequently have to write. Then we'll show you an example of a formal analytical report that uses a number of topic headings and statistical support in the form of graphs and tables.

SELF-EVALUATION REPORTS

A self-evaluation report describes what you were able to accomplish over a given period of time. It is often requested as part of a yearly performance evaluation (see Chapter 7). As you climb the management ladder, your job descriptions will typically become less specific. This means that you have more freedom to be creative with your time, but it also means that you may be accountable for how you spend that time.

The best way to write a self-evaluation report is to be prepared to do it. It's obvious that in order to report on progress, you have to know where you started and where you expected to end. In other words, write objectives (see Chapter 6). In the interim, keep records of your accomplishments. It's also a good idea to make notes about snags that you encountered which forced you to abandon or redefine your objectives. The report is not difficult to write if you follow these suggestions. In addition, this approach will demonstrate to your boss that you are organized and effective in your job. It may also help you to draft realistic objectives for the next year. Here is an example of a self-evaluation report submitted by a newly appointed clinical specialist at the request of the director of nursing.

As we discussed after my appointment last month, I would report on my activities as a clinical specialist by September 30. As you will recall, my objectives for this first month were the following:

1. Draft a job description for an oncology clinical specialist.

2. Begin to establish the role of clinical specialist for oncology patients.

The job description was drafted and submitted to the Nursing Practice Council on September 15. I have not yet received notice of Council's action.

I have begun to establish the role of oncology clinical specialist through the following activities:

1. Conferred with the area supervisor, nursing staff, medical staff, and patient support services to introduce the role of a clinical nurse specialist.

2. Participated in the care and support of three terminally ill patients and their families. This is part of role-modeling for nursing staff and is addressed in the job description.

3. Presented an inservice program on the CBC and Differential at the request of nursing staff.

4. Surveyed nurses who care for oncology patients to find out their continuing education interests and needs. As a result of this survey, I am planning an education series on the leukemias for next month.

One recurring theme in my conference with staff and physicians is the need to designate one unit as the oncology unit. I would like to discuss this further with you when we meet later this week. At that time, I will also present to you my objectives for next month.

As you read this report were you able to determine its purpose? Was it clear, interesting, and thorough? Compare the previous report with this one:

Date: September 30, 1985

To: Jane Nichols

From: John Barber

Re: Self-Evaluation

I am happy to report that I am making good progress in my clinical specialist role. I have almost completed the draft of my job description. In addition, I have met with several people to discuss my role and found them to be supportive. Based on these discussions, I am confident that I will be able to provide a much-needed service for oncology patients.

While this example may still qualify as a self-evaluation report, it is too general and biased to be of much value. If you were the boss, which report would you rather receive?

STATISTICAL REPORTS

Part of your job as a nurse manager may require that you gather data and present it in an organized manner. While most of us cringe at the thought of statistics, they are useful in analyzing data in preparation for decision making. Generally speaking, the reports that you will be writing will not require the use of the more complex statistical tests but will only require that you learn to use descriptive statistics.

Descriptive Measures

Two frequently used descriptive measures are the mean and percentage. The mean is one of the measures of central tendency; it is the average of a group of figures. A percentage is a calculation which shows how much of 100 a certain number is. Using these two descriptive measures accurately will probably meet most of your statistical reporting needs.

CALCULATING A MEAN

The mean is the average of a group of figures. To find the mean, add all of the figures in the column and divide by the total number of figures. For example, find the average number (mean) of overtime hours worked in the intensive care units in a week based on the following data: MICU, 5 hours; SICU, 17 hours; Coronary Care, 3 hours. Your answer should be 8.3 hours. (Add 5, 17, and 3; divide by 3.)

This example also points out one of the dangers of calculating a mean. It may hide very large or very small numbers. In the case cited, it might be more meaningful to examine the overtime trends over a period of time to find out if SICU overtime is always that high.

CALCULATING A PERCENTAGE

Converting numbers to a percentage of 100 provides a basis for comparing numbers that are not alike. When expressed as a percentage of 100, numbers may be more meaningful. For example, if 13 nurses in MICU, 7 from SICU, and 23 from the medical-surgical units hold bachelor's degrees, it appears as though more nurses from the med-surg units hold degrees. However, when calculated as percentages it might be that 86.6% (13 of 15) of MICU nurses, 58.3% (7 of 12) of SICU nurses, and 31.9% (23 of 72 nurses) of med-surg nurses hold bachelor's degrees. This result is markedly different from the real numbers expressed first.

Percentages are calculated by first expressing the numbers as a fraction and then multiplying by 100. As cited above, the percentage of MICU nurses holding bachelor's degrees was obtained by dividing 13 (number holding degrees) by 15 (total number of nurses in MICU). The result, .866, was then mulipied by 100 to obtain 86.6%.

A word of caution is also important here. The comparison of numbers converted into percentages is valid only if the size of the groups being compared is approximately the same. There is a risk of distortion when comparing two unlike groups.

Organizing Data

When presenting numbers in the body of a report, you will want to organize it so that the reader will be able to understand it clearly. Two common ways of summarizing and organizing data are tables and graphs. Remember that presenting data in tables and graphs does not substitute for analysis in the narrative. A table or graph should illustrate or enhance the written description, not replace it.

USE OF TABLES

A Table allows for the presentation of numerical data in columns and rows. This method of organization allows your reader to better understand how the numbers are related and will often make your report more clear.

General rules for constructing tables are:

1. Write the title carefully so that it tells the reader exactly what the table is about.
2. Keep variables or categories of information to a minimum.
3. Name each row and column so that the reader can identify what variables are being presented.
4. If percentages are used, cite both the number and the percentage.
5. Tables should be internally consistent:
   a. Percentages should add up to 100, or you should explain why they do not.
   b. Be sure that addition is correct if numbers in columns are totalled.

USE OF GRAPHS

A graph is a picture of a comparison of variables. Its purposes, like that of a table, are to clarify relationships for the reader and to enhance the written description. There are two basic types of graphs: line graphs and bar graphs.

Line Graphs.   Line graphs are constructed on two axes. The y-axis is vertical, the x-axis horizontal. The line of the graph represents the relationship between two variables (x and y). If one variable is time, it is usually placed in the x-axis, while frequency is most usually shown on the y-axis. Values of each variable are plotted on the graph and then connected by a line. The line indicates the general trend of the relationship between variables. A good example of a line graph is the temperature graph used to indicate patients' temperatures, which presents patterns much more clearly than a list of temperature recordings.

Bar Graphs.   Bar graphs are used to compare several categories on one dimension. Bars may be drawn either horizontally or vertically. Each bar must be carefully labeled to make the relationships clear. As with line graphs and tables, bar graphs do not substitute for a written description of the data.

A Sample Statistical Report

Suppose you were asked by your boss to summarize the performance of graduate nurses employed during a six-month period. The purpose of the summary report is to compare the performance of graduate nurses of different educational backgrounds and make recomendations for future hiring and hospital orientation procedures. The example which follows contains:

1. An Introduction
2. A Presentation of Data
3. An Analysis of Data
4. A Discussion
5. Conclusions and Recommendations

Performance of Graduate Professional Nurses Employed January to July, 1985

Introduction

The purpose of this study is to determine the level of performance of graduate nurses at three and six months according to type of professional education. The results of this study may identify a significant area for consideration in selecting and orienting employees.

All graduate professional nurses are rated by the head nurse of the clinical unit at three months and six months after employement. The "Registered Nurse Performance Appraisal" is the evaluation tool. Using these evaluations to collect data required no change in the usual evaluation procedures of the institution, and therefore was not time consuming or costly.

The limitations of this method are that the raters (head nurses of the clinical units) are not controlled, the scale used in rating the performance contains subjective terminology, and there is no measure of baseline performance of the graduate nurses.

The Registered Nurse Performance Appraisal contains 40 behavior-oriented statements for which the evaluator is asked to score the nurse's performance according to the following scale:

1. No evidence of performance.
2. Performance variable.
3. Criteria usually met, needs occasional guidance.
4. Criteria met consistently.
5. Usually exceeds expectations.

All data reported reflect the use of this 5-point scale.

To aid in the analysis of data, the criteria on the performance appraisal form were divided into three categories according to the following definitions:

I. Technical Skill (15 items): procedures/behaviors that involve performance of a "task"; synthesis of knowledge or thought processes are a significant part of this behavior.

II. Interpersonal Relationships (15 items): behaviors that primarily involve communication skills.

III. Personal/Professional Responsibility Behaviors (10 items): behaviors that measure or indicate a sense of responsibility/accountability to self, others, the institution, or the nursing profession.

The population sample of 62 newly graduated professional nurses consisted of 8 nurses prepared at the Baccalaureate level (BSN), 46 nurses prepared in diploma schools (DIPL), and 8 nurses prepared in Associate Degree (AD) programs.

Mean Performance Scores

At three months, the BSN had the lowest mean performance score at 2.91, the AD was next highest at 3.01, while the DIPL nurses showed the best mean performance at 3.19. The performance scores at six months show the AD lowest (3.15), DIPL next (3.34), and the BSN highest (3.36). Note that the performance of the AD at six months is slightly behind that of the DIPL at three months. Table 1 contains mean performance scores for each of the three groups and percentage of improvement from three to six months. The percentage of improvement for the DIPL group is lowest, followed by the AD group, and the BSN group, whose percentage of improvement is substantially higher.

Table 1   Mean Performance Scores at Three and Six Months and Percentage of Improvement by Education

Education	3 Month	6 Month	% Improvement
AD	3.01	3.26	8.3%
DIPL	3.19	3.34	4.7%
BSN	2.91	3.36	15.5%

Analysis of Performance by Category

Analysis of performance scores for each category at three months reveals the same pattern as the overall scores: BSN lowest, AD next, and DIPL highest. However, at six months, the BSN scored second highest in Technical Skills and Professional Responsibility and highest in Interpersonal Relationships. Table 2 contains performance scores for each group according to the three categories of performance. The greatest percentage of improvement in any one category between three months and six months was demonstrated by the BSN nurses in the Interpersonal Relationships category (22.9%). The rate of improvement in Category II (Interpersonal Relationships) for AD and DIPL nurses lags behind the rate of improvement in Technical and Professional Responsibility. Of note also in Table 2 is that the scores for Professional Responsibility behaviors at six months for all educational levels are within .05 points of each other. Figure 1 graphically shows the improvement of graduate nurses according to education and category of behavior. Note the rapid rate of improvement of the BSN nurses.

Discussion

Significant points to be considered in the discussion of these results are the orientation program and method of classification for each of the three groups. Currently, all graduate nurses enter at the same level and are classified as Level I. After six months they are eligible for transfer to permanent status or Level II. During the six-month time period each nurse receives a formal orientation program. The formal orientation for Diploma and BSN nurses is 6 weeks in length while that of the AD nurse is 12 weeks or twice as long. With this information in mind, the following points and questions should be considered:

1. The results raise a question about the justification for the double orientation costs of the AD graduate nurse. However, it is important to recognize the lack of *control* of evaluators and the possibility of subconscious prejudice against the AD graduate and her performance.

Table 2 Performance Score According to Category

	Technical Skill			Interpersonal Relationship			Professional Responsibility		
	3 Mo.	6 Mo.	%	3 Mo.	6 Mo.	%	3 Mo.	6 Mo.	%
AD	2.92	3.22	10.3	2.96	3.16	6.8	3.15	3.40	7.9
DIPL	3.12	3.33	7.0	3.15	3.23	2.5	3.28	3.45	5.2
BSN	2.88	3.24	12.5	2.80	3.44	22.9	3.04	3.40	11.8
Mean	2.97	3.26	9.0	2.97	3.28	9.5	3.16	3.42	7.7

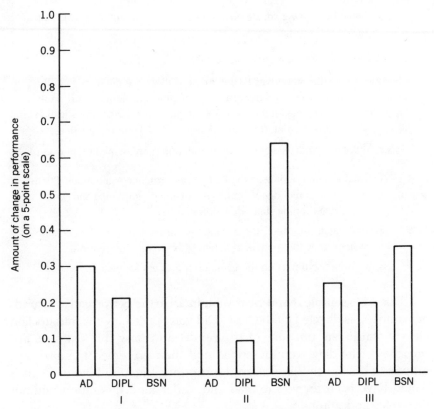

Figure 5.1. Improvement of graduate nurse performance from three months to six months according to level of education and category of behavior measured.

2. The level of performance of the BSN nurses at three months may raise serious doubts about their effectiveness. However, these doubts are erased by their superior performance at six months. This factor reaffirms the need for a six-month probationary period for this group.

3. Further investigation is needed to determine if the rate of growth betwen three and six months is a predictor of rate of growth between six months and one year. When, if ever, does performance plateau? Does the fact that there are no promotions between Level II and the Assistant Head Nurse position influence rate of growth after six months?

4. What correlation, if any, exists between performance evaluations during the educational process and practice as a professional nurse?

5. Should the new graduate nurses be classified according to education level?

Conclusions and Recommendations

The purpose of this study was to determine if there are differences in the level of performance of graduate nurses of differing educational backgrounds. The results suggest this may be true. However, further investigation is necessary before this information can be applied to hiring practices.

As a result of this study, several recommendations can be made. They are:

1. Establish an ongoing analysis of all performance evaluations. Such a program could identify trends in nursing performance and be useful in determining staff education needs.

2. Investigate the need for expanding the present job classification system to accommodate a system of horizontal promotion.

3. Conduct seminars on the evaluation process for evaluators.

   Does this sample report clearly summarize the performance of graduate nurses, as directed by the boss? Did you notice how the introduction clearly stated the purpose of the report and how the task was approached? The data were described and then presented in tables and graphs to enchance the written description. Imagine how difficult it would have been for you to read and understand this report without the tables and graphs.

   A discussion of the results and conclusions and recommendations are often useful to include. However, they may not be necessary in all statistical reports. You can decide whether or not to include these based on the expectations of your reader. In this case, the writer felt comfortable sharing his or her ideas about the results with the reader. It's important to note, however, that the reader might interpret the results differently and reach other conclusions.

CRITICAL INCIDENT REPORTS

Many institutions have standardized forms for reporting critical incidents and policies which specify what needs to be reported and to whom.

However, on these forms there is usually a section where the nurse must describe the incident.

When reporting a critical incident such as a patient fall or medication error, it is important to present the facts of the incident in a clear and organized manner. Further, you should be certain that you present enough information so that if you need to refer to it at a future date the incident will be clear in your mind. A good way to check on the clarity of your description is to have someone read it who was uninvolved in the incident. Ask the person to be critical of your description and to consider what additional information may be needed.

Be careful to present only *factual* material which may have contributed to or resulted from the incident. Your description should never contain opinions or conclusions. Consider the examples that follow. Which one is clear and factual? (Assume that the patient's age, diagnosis, physician, date, time, etc. are recorded elsewhere on the form report.)

> Mr. Jones was found on the floor of his room. He was apparently confused and climbed out of bed to use the bathroom. He was helped to his feet and assisted back to bed. His vital signs were stable and he is not complaining of injury.

> Mr. Jones was found lying on the floor of his room. When questioned, he stated that he was trying to get to the bathroom. He received a sedative at midnight and was sleeping in bed with siderails up at 1:00 a.m. nursing rounds. His call bell was attached to the left siderail. The vital signs taken previous to the incident were at 10:00 p.m. (BP 128/88, P 76). Vital signs after the incident were BP 130/90, P 86. He denies pain; however, inspection of the skin reveals a one-inch bruise of the right knee and a thumbnail-sized abrasion of the left elbow. He was assisted back to bed and instructed to call for assistance if he needs to get up again. There were no witnesses to the incident.

Note that the second example is factual and clearly written. It also indicates the status of the patient before and after the fall. The nurse who wrote the first example might have real difficulty recalling the details of the incident several weeks or months later. The nurse who wrote the second could refer to this description as written and feel confident that Mr. Jones was cared for properly.

MINUTES OF MEETINGS

When you call a meeting, you should be certain that someone is assigned to record the proceedings of the meeting. This written record of business conducted at a meeting serves to remind participants of tasks assigned to them, decisions reached by the group, and information that was circulated. In addition, minutes provide a reference for persons unable to attend the meeting.

Begin by recording the title of the group and the date, time, and location of the meeting. A list of participants and those who should have been present but were not is a useful tool for the circulation of the minutes and is included as part of the heading.

Minutes should be kept as brief as possible while still conveying the essential information. If parliamentary procedure is followed, the minutes can be organized around those headings. If not, organize your notes according to topics covered. It is not necessary to record verbatim what is said, as long as what you record reflects the essence of any discussions. Motions made should be recorded accurately as well as the outcome of the vote. This is also true for decisions made by the group or tasks assigned to members of the group. In most cases, an outline format provides an adequate record of proceedings and is easily read. Minutes should end with a notation of the time of adjournment and the date and time of the next meeting.

A common misuse of minutes that should be avoided is the tendency to use them as a substitute for circulating information outside of the group. Decisions made by the group which affect others must be communicated more formally to those affected. This might be done effectively through a memo, a letter, or a report.

6

Writing Effective Objectives

An integral part of the management process is the ability to write objectives. Simply described, an objective is a precise statement of what needs to be accomplished, by whom, in what manner, and in what period of time. Well thought out and effectively written objectives can be a valuable tool for self-direction of your managerial activities.

When you are asked by higher level managers to write objectives, it forces you to assess your present situation carefully and define what may need to be changed in order for you to effectively carry out the purposes, philosophy, and goals of your institution. In addition, setting objectives helps a manager focus energy toward a specific activity or group of activities. This can help you avoid getting stalled in the daily troubleshooting activities present in any nurse manager's job. Finally, well-defined objectives provide a fair basis for evaluation of your performance as a manager. (See Chapter 7 for more information on performance evaluation.)

THE NEED FOR OBJECTIVES

The push in health care institutions toward a management by objectives system grew out of the work of Peter Drucker, who described the concept in the 1950s. The system was designed to improve the motivation and productivity of the worker by obtaining worker participation in goal setting. It has proved useful in many health care institutions, because the daily high stress environment can completely consume a manager's time and energy, leaving little time for improving delivery of patient care.

Many nurse managers feel initial resentment when faced with the task of writing objectives. These feelings grow out of the fact that it is difficult to see beyond day-to-day stresses to long-term goals. There seems little enough time to deal with today's crises, let alone look months ahead. However, we can argue that focusing at least part of the manager's attention beyond immediate concerns provides an opportunity for long-range improvements. In addition, when you have specific objectives that must be accomplished in a certain time, you will be forced to delegate responsibility to subordinates, which may also prepare them for future managerial assignments.

Critics of management by objectives believe that the system may stifle creativity by forcing people to concentrate their energies in too narrow a scope. A well-run system, however, might include opportunities to renegotiate or redefine objectives as situations change. Any system that is applied too rigidly seems doomed to failure, but management by objectives can be flexible and creative.

Managers at all levels of the institutional hierarchy need to perceive that their superiors agree with and are committed to objectives that have been established. In certain cases, this support may require the commitment of funds in order to carry out the program effectively. Such support can be established and maintained through interaction and feedback among appropriate levels of management. The most successful systems stem from strong top management groups that have well-defined institutional goals and purposes. Often these are longer range and less detailed than specific objectives. However, they must be carefully selected in order to reflect the need for improvement or change in the current situation. Each succeeding level in the management hierarchy can then be charged with determining specifically how the general goals will be carried out.

A final and very important element in an effective system of management by objectives is wide participation in the process. When people are asked to participate in defining and refining goals and objectives, they will probably be more committed to carrying them out than when the goals and objectives are dictated from above. This does not mean that top management cannot define direction, only that direction is more effective when all parties involved participate in shaping that direction.

You may be asked to write two general types of objectives: *personal* and *institutional*. Personal objectives are statements about the need for change or improvement on a personal level. For example, a head nurse may have determined that he or she is ineffective at leading group discussions of unit personnel. The problem having been identified, she or he could draft a specific objective to improve this element of management. Defining and using personal objectives is an integral part of employee performance evaluation, and we will discuss the process in detail in Chapter 7.

Organizational objectives, which we will discuss in this chapter, relate to specific areas or aspects of the institution that are targeted for change or improvement. All organizational objectives should derive from the purposes, philosopy, and goals of the institution. To illustrate how these organizational objectives might be identified and written, we will use the following sample case throughout this chapter.

A SAMPLE CASE

Imagine that the statement of purpose of our sample institution contains the following sentence: *The overall purpose of this health care institution is to provide quality health care for its clients.* The institution's philosophy further states, *The health care that is received by a client is based on health needs and not on socioeconomic situation.* The director of nursing and a group of supervisors are beginning to realize that there is room for improvement in the quality of health care that patients are receiving. They have discussed the situation extensively and have decided that the present system of team nursing is outdated and is contributing to stagnation in the delivery of quality patient care. After careful consideration of institutional purpose, philosophy, and goals, they decide to implement a primary nursing system.

A long-range goal developed for the department states that the system be operational in two years, with the first year devoted to planning, revision of policies and procedures, and staff education. The second year will involve gradual implementation of the system on a unit-by-unit basis to allow time for management of change conflict and troubleshooting. (The time schedule must always be carefully considered because, if unrealistic, it will contribute to the failure of the objective.)

With the establishment of these deparmental objectives, each subordinate's group within the department must now draft objectives to define their role in implementing the new system.

THE MECHANICS OF WRITING OBJECTIVES

Workable, effective objectives are statements of who will do what, in what manner, by what time. They also contain "action" verbs so that they can be easily evaluated. The long-range departmental goal described in the example might look like this:

> By January 1, 1987 the department of nursing will implement a primary nursing system on all nursing units.

You can further define tasks and clarify actions in the following manner:

> During 1985, in preparation for the conversion to a primary nursing system:
>
> 1. The assistant directors of nursing will review and revise the policy and procedure manuals in preparation for conversion to primary nursing.
> 2. The staff development department will design and implement a program to educate staff nurses in the mechanics of the primary nursing system.
> 3. After attending the education program, the head nurse of each unit will submit a report on the feasibility of implementing the primary nursing system on a particular unit.

These very specific objectives leave little doubt as to who will be doing what in the coming year. Notice the use of action verbs such as *implement, revise, design,* and *submit*. These words clearly define what will be done and can be easily evaluated. If the persons carrying out the objective do not implement, revise, design, or submit, then the objective has not been met. To further illustrate this point, suppose the staff development department's objective stated "To raise the level of knowledge and understanding of unit personnel regarding the primary nursing system." Why is this objective less effective than the one stated previously? How is the level of knowledge and understanding measured? How will this task be accomplished? While this objective may sound fancier and contain bigger words, it is less effective because it does not clearly define who will do what, in what manner, by what time. Remember the most effective objectives are those which are stated simply and clearly.

STARTING FROM SCRATCH

What happens when there is no specific departmental project outlined for you to focus objectives on, but as part of your job you are asked to submit objectives for the coming year? While this makes the task a little more difficult, it is not impossible. An advantage in this situation is that you can focus objectives on areas that are of personal interest or that need special attention within your area of control. The following steps outline what to do when starting from scratch:

1. Conduct a thorough assessment of the situation. These questions will help you get started: What is the current status of patient care in my areas? What is the level of patient satisfaction? What is the level of personnel satisfaction? Are staffing turnover or assignments a problem? Are personnel up-to-date on current information in their area of specialty? Are reference resources adequate? Is the nursing process utilized effectively? Do personnel conform to policies or procedures? What are the current issues in nursing that may affect my personnel?

2. Review your personal job description. What areas do you perform effectively? What areas do you need to improve?

3. Prioritize the items on your list. Which are directly related to institutional philosophy, purpose, or objectives? Which items are most important to your subordinates? Which items are most important or interesting to you? What resources might be needed

to change these problem areas? Which items can be accomplished in a reasonable amount of time?

4. Share your findings with another manager on your level or discuss them with your immediate supervisor.

5. Draft specific objectives designed to meet the areas of need that you have identified. It might also be helpful to include a statement for each objective as to why this particular objective is important.

Suppose that you are the head nurse of a recently established oncology unit. One of the recurring problems that you notice is that your staff have difficulty understanding the reasons why certain treatment regimens are prescribed by physicians. You feel that there is a need for improved communication among nursing staff and physicians. In addition, you realize that the patient would benefit if all members of the health care team were well informed about specific patient situations and medical needs. You decide to incorporate the assessed need as one of your objectives to be accomplished the following year. Based on this situation, the objective you draft might look like this:

> To establish a weekly patient care conference for members of the oncology health care team.

Once you have drafted your objective, you may need to "sell" it to your supervisor. This selling process would include a description of why the objective is important (need), who will be involved in the implementation, how the objective will be implemented, when this will occur, and whether or not it will require money, personnel, or equipment. By anticipating and answering the questions that your boss might have related to your objective, you will increase the chances of it being accepted.

SUMMARY

Writing objectives is an important part of every nurse manager's job. Well-written objectives help to organize the work load of the manager and lead to a sense of accomplishment when they have been satisfied. In addition, they serve as excellent documentation of the nurse manager's performance. For these reasons, it is important that you learn to write objectives effectively.

7

Performance
Evaluations

Evaluating the performance of a subordinate is undoubtedly the least
favorite task of the nurse manager. Some factors which make this task
unpleasant include poor manager training, ineffective and nonexisting
evaluation instruments, and reluctance to confront a poorly performing
subordinate. Performance evaluation is an integral part of organizational
decision making and the realization of organizational goals; therefore,
it must be effectively conducted.

What is the purpose of evaluation? How is it conducted? How often
should a subordinate be evaluated? What is good performance? Poor
performance? These and other questions are common among all types
of managers and are stumbling blocks in the evaluation process. This
chapter is devoted to demystifying the evaluation process and helping
you to write more effective evaluations.

PURPOSE

The general purpose of an evaluation is to determine how well a subordinate is doing his or her job. The outcome of the evaluation may

indicate a need for extra guidance or training to improve performance or indicate a readiness for promotion. On a broader scale, the evaluation process can serve as a measure of how well the mission of the institution is being carried out and indicate problem areas that need to be addressed in organizational objectives, policies, or procedures. Consider the following example.

Nancy S., supervisor of the surgical units in a large metropolitan hospital, received a report from the nurse epidemiologist that the rate of postsurgical wound infections was significantly lower in one unit than in the others under her control. During a performance evaluation conference with Bob Z., the head nurse of the unit, Nancy discovered that Bob had initiated an infection awareness program on his unit after observing several breaks in sterile technique by his personnel. Nancy asked Bob to share his program with the staff development instructor so that it could be used throughout the hospital.

In this example, the head nurse discovered a nursing care problem during observation of personnel, an important step in the performance evaluation process. The supervisor shared her favorable report from the epidemiologist and discovered that the head nurse had recognized a problem and taken the appropriate steps to solve it. This is an important and easily documented example of how well the head nurse is performing, and one that might be used in Bob's favor in deciding promotability or wage increases. On the other units, the supervisor could indicate to the head nurses that postsurgical infections were higher than expected and ask them to identify and solve the problem. Their success during this task could indicate how well they are performing as head nurses and perhaps indicate a need for increased guidance.

Performance is evaluated by outcomes and observation. During this measurement, performance is compared with others of the same level or a set of predetermined criteria (outcome) and a rating or judgment is made. The results of this rating form an important basis for employee development, administrative decision making, and planning. The performance evaluation process is closely related to the organization's mission, a fact that makes it one of your most important tasks.

THE EVALUATION PROCESS

Understanding the evaluation process will make your job of writing an evaluation much easier. Many managers find themselves faced with a set of performance evaluations that are due to be written and they don't know where to begin. The difficulty may lie in the lack of understanding of the purposes and components of the evaluation process. Every evaluation should be approached with this question in your mind: How well is this employee doing his or her job? The answers to this question cannot be left until the actual writing of the report; rather, it must be a question foremost in your mind at all times. The written evaluation is a summary of the evaluation process and *not* the process in itself.

The steps in the evaluation process are:

1. Direct observation of the subordinate's performance and/or observation of the outcomes of performance.
2. Comparison of job performance with specific criteria for performance.
3. Documentation of critical incidents.
4. Translation of these observations and comparisons onto an evaluation instrument.
5. Presentation to the employee.
6. Mutual goal setting for the next evaluation period.

We will discuss each of these steps in the sections that follow.

Observation of Performance And/Or Outcomes

The most objective method of performance evaluation is direct observation of the employee while he or she is functioning on the job. This does not imply that the employee should be shadowed by the evaluator. This would threaten or produce anxiety and might, therefore, negatively affect the employee's performance. Rather, the evaluator should take every opportunity to participate with the employee during job performance and thus observe the employee in action. Some examples include:

1. Making rounds with head nurses and observing the way they communicate with and assess patients.
2. Attending a patient care conference conducted by a staff nurse.
3. Assisting and observing a licensed practical nurse caring for a multiproblem patient.

This direct observation can be accomplished at an informal level by recognizing employee evaluation as an ongoing process instead of something that is done intermittently.

Another objective way to evaluate is to look at the outcomes of the employee's performance. The example about postoperative infection rate described earlier illustrates the use of outcomes. Others include:

1. Patient comments, both positive and negative.
2. Complaints or lack of complaints from co-workers.
3. Incident reports involving omission and commission errors during practice.
4. Audit review of patient charts and nursing care plans.

Performance Criteria

Effective evaluation is impossible unless expectations of performance are clearly written. The most logical basis for evaluation is the job description, which can be expanded or clarified through written standards of performance and personal and organizational objectives. A subordinate cannot perform effectively or be evaluated fairly unless you spell out expectations for performance. This is illustrated by the following example:

Joe S. had just completed his orientation as a nurse aide. One of his assigned duties was to take and record the a.m. TPRs of the patients in his unit. Joe counted Mr. N.'s pulse as 130 at 8:00 a.m. and recorded it on the TPR worksheet. At 10:00 a.m., the head nurse noticed that Mr. N. looked pale and tired. She counted his pulse and discovered the high rate. She immediately notified the physician and Mr. N. was transferred to a monitored bed. The head nurse then called Joe in to discuss the incident. Joe stated that he had understood his duty to be to take and record the TPR. He was not aware of the need to report abnormalities to anyone and indeed the nurse aide's job description stated only "take and record TPRs."

Perhaps a more experienced aide would have recognized the potential danger in this situation, but it was unfair to expect Joe to do so.

Documentation of Critical Incidents

Another part of the evaluation process is documentation of critical incidents. Once again, the information you gather and document before writing the evaluation is most important. Perhaps the reasons so many managers dislike evaluation is that they do not have concrete information available when it comes time to actually write the final copy. A way to remedy this is to keep a log of the performance of each of your subordinates. The log should contain information about specific incidents related to performance. For example:

6/28/83   Ann left the unit without completing the narcotics count for the a.m. shift. Counseled 6/29/83.

7/15/83   Ann worked 4 hrs. overtime due to shortstaffing.

9/01/83   Called away 1 hr. early due to illness of child.

9/20/83   Assumed charge responsibilities in absence of head nurse. She performed well, except for misquoting the hospital visiting policy to a family member which resulted in a complaint by the family to the administrator. After discussion with Ann, I believe that she was not appropriately informed by the head nurse of the change in hospital policy. Ann agreed to review the visiting policy.

These very specific notes can be a tremendous aid to you in writing the final evaluation. Not only do they help you to complete a fair evaluation, but they are useful in demonstrating to the employee specific instances of good and not-so-good performance. A sensible rule of thumb for evaluation is that if the rating is above or below average, it should be accompanied by an explanation. This documentation is equally important in employee promotion and dismissal, and you can avoid serious problems for yourself and your institution if you use it.

TIPS FOR WRITING CRITICAL INCIDENT NOTES

1. Never write the note the same day as the incident, especially if it is a negative note. You will be more objective the next day.

2. Write the note while the incident is fresh in your mind.

3. Keep notes consistently.

4. Write both positive and negative notes; all positive or all negative notes will color your evaluation.

5. Be sure the notes are specific enough to trigger your memory. This is especially important for annual evaluations.

6. Keep these notes to yourself. They should not be typed by a secretary or seen by other personnel.

The Evaluation Tool

Many institutions use a rating scale approach to employee evaluation. This was adopted in an attempt to simplify the evaluation process. The difficulty with this is twofold: the evaluation is not simple, and these rating scales are often too general to be of much use. The Joint Commission on the Accreditation of Hospitals has recommended that evaluation of nursing personnel be criteria-based, that is, that evaluation criteria be generated from philosophy, objectives, and job descriptions.

In the absence of specific rating criteria, you can seek ways to use a general form more effectively. For example, initiative and dependability are common employee characteristics found on general rating forms. Consider how these characteristics differ according to levels of personnel, such as a staff nurse, a licensed practical nurse, and a nurse aide. What areas of the job description are related to these characteristics? Be sure to give specific examples of the employee's initiative and dependability or lack of them. These examples will help to further clarify expectations and aid the employee in improving performance.

A good evaluation instrument contains specific statements about performance that are easily rated. Here are some examples from a staff nurse evaluation:

1. Obtains a comprehensive health history.

2. Develops and updates a comprehensive patient care plan.

3. Administers medications safely.

With this type of form, your job then is to elaborate what is meant by "comprehensive health history" and give specific guidance to the staff nurses to help improve their performance.

Consider the following evaluation statements. Why are these less useful than those listed previously?

1. Understands the care planning process.

2. Has knowledge of safe medication administration.

3. Shows initiative.

If you decided that 1 and 2 are not behavioral performance statements, and that 3 is not easily defined or explained, you were right.

In summary, the ideal form for evaluation of performance would contain specific statements, easily measured and explained, and related to the job description. In the absence of this type of instrument, you should be prepared to elaborate on the employee's job description and the existing tool so that the evaluation process can be meaningful for the employee and the institution.

Many performance evaluation instruments are accompanied by a rating scale to help quantify the employee's performance. The difficulty with a scale containing four or more choices is that inflation tends to occur. One way to avoid inflation is to adopt a two-point scale for the criteria:

2: meets criteria

1: does not consistently meet criteria

The problem with this scale is that persons who perform beyond what is expected will be hidden among those who are performing adequately. Adding a third category (3: *consistently does more than is expected*) and requiring a supporting statement for a rating of 3 or 1 will separate out the best and the worst from the average. In addition, the 3 category may serve as a motivation for some employees to improve their performance and demonstrate the potential for promotion.

Presentation To The Employee

This aspect is equally important in ensuring an effective evaluation outcome. The written evaluation, job description, and performance standards should be given to the subordinate at least two days before the evaluation conference. This gives the person being evaluated an opportunity to review the evaluation in private and think about its contents. If there is a negative emotional reaction, this previewing will give the employee time to sort out and control feelings and to be better able to discuss the evaluation rationally. Remember that the primary focus of evaluation is not reward/punishment, but rather a means of motivating an employee to improved performance. In many instances, it is helpful to have the employee complete a self-evaluation (before reading your evaluation) which is submitted to you for review before the conference. In this way, both employee and manager have input in the process and each can see the position of the other. Ideally, the self-evaluation and your evaluation would not differ significantly. If they do, then you need to focus on these differences in the evaluation conference.

Mutual Goal Setting

The employee should emerge from the evaluation conference with a list of goals/objectives to guide performance for the next rating period. The goals should focus on areas of performance that need improvement, participation in organizational goals, or professional development of the employee. To be effective in motivating performance, the goals should be mutually determined. However, in the case of a poorly performing employee, you may need to set goals for the employee to meet during the next evaluation period. You may also request that the subordinate submit a plan for meeting the objectives at a later date. This may increase the motivation of the subordinate to meet the goals.

Consider the following examples of goals for a ward clerk, a staff nurse, and a head nurse. Are they clearly defined, easily measured?

1. Goal: To arrive at the workplace on or before the scheduled time.
   Plan: I will contact the Personnel Director for information on car pools from my area.

2. Goal: To write a comprehensive care plan on each of my primary patients within 24 hours of admission.

   Plan: Contact the staff development instructor for help in constructing the care plan.

3. Goal: To use the appropriate procedure for employee disciplinary action.

   Plan: (a) I will review the hospital policy and procedure related to employee disciplinary action.

   (b) I will attend the staff development seminar entitled "Dealing with Problem Staff."

   (c) I will contact my supervisor for guidance before approaching the next employee with a disciplinary problem.

LEGAL ASPECTS OF PERFORMANCE EVALUATION

The creation of the Federal Equal Employment Opportunity Commission has motivated many organizations to "clean up their act" relative to personnel decision making, and has given employees the right to challenge personnel decisions. The following situations are illustrations of two common employee relation problems that are closely related to performance evaluation.

Case 1

Joe S., the nurse's aide discussed previously in the chapter, was fired shortly after the incident with Mr. N. He feels that he was treated unfairly by you because of a personality conflict, and he has decided to appeal to the hospital administrator.

Case 2

Sue J. expected to be promoted to evening supervisor because she was the head nurse with the most experience. You promoted John L. instead. Sue decides to complain about her unfair treatment to the Director of Nursing and has threatened to hire a lawyer.

The questions listed below are examples of the kind of information your superiors will need in order to decide whether to support or reverse your decision.

1. Were the policies and procedures of the institution followed? Examples of policies and procedures that might apply in these situations are frequency and conduct of performance evaluations, disciplinary action, probation, and termination.
2. Were the performance evaluations valid and reliable?
    (a) Validity means that the evaluations are actually measuring what they are supposed to measure—job performance. A poorly constructed evaluation instrument could be legally challenged and declared invalid. This is true especially in the case of those evaluation instruments that are not clearly job-related or where job descriptions and performance criteria are vague or nonexistent.
    (b) Reliability refers to the way in which the actual rating is done. Theoretically, two raters with similar experience should rate the performance of an employee similarly if they were using the same instrument and observed the employee at the same time. This is referred to as interrater reliability. Another type of reliability is intrarater; that is, the rating would be the same if performed on two consecutive days by the same person. In other words, the rater has to be careful not to let extraneous factors such as hunger, headache, or time of day influence the rating. A third type of reliability has to do with the purpose of the evaluation. In order to be considered reliable, the rating would be the same whether it was being used for promotion, merit increases, or employee development.
3. Is there documentation accompanying the rating?
4. Were the employees fully aware of performance expectations? How were these communicated? Is there documentation to this effect?
5. Were the performance ratings completed and presented to the employees in an appropriate manner?

If the above questions could be answered affirmatively, then your superior should support your decision, and you should feel confident that you have prepared a defensible performance evaluation.

SUMMARY

The central purpose of performance evaluation is to determine how well an employee is doing a job. This information can be further used for employee development, as a basis for administrative decision making, and to indicate how well the mission of the institution is being carried out.

A successful and meaningful performance evaluation process "hangs together ; that is, it is derived from organizational philosophy and objectives which are expanded into individual job descriptions. Performance standards and evaluation criteria are then derived from these descriptions. Employees are rated, counseled, and asked to participate in drawing up objectives and plans to improve performance.

By following the steps outlined in this chapter, you can make a valuable contribution to employee development and organizational mission.

SUMMARY

8

Guidelines for Writing Policies and Procedures

The general purpose of policy and procedure manuals is to provide a framework for day-to-day operation of the health care institution. This framework promotes organization and consistency, and helps to prevent conflict and chaos. Well-written policy and procedure manuals can facilitate more effective use of the nurse manager's time by freeing the manager from overseeing routine activities.

Policy and procedure manuals must be taken seriously by all involved parties including top management. New employees should be required to review manuals as part of their job orientation. Commonly, though, these manuals are dust collectors. They are not used consistently usually because they are poorly written, out-of-date, or so disorganized that they are impossible to use readily.

This chapter will outline some general guidelines for writing policies and procedures and then describe the specific differences between them. By following the guidelines suggested here, you can make policy and procedure manuals more effective and promote their use.

111

GENERAL POINTS TO CONSIDER

Effective policies and procedures must be clearly stated in writing and contained in a common, accessible place. Often, memos are used to announce changes in policies and procedures, but these must be followed by a comprehensive statement of policy or a detailed procedure to be placed in their respective manuals. A memo is not a suitable replacement for these because it is too easily lost or forgotten.

The organization of the manuals is extremely important. Three-ring binders are very useful in that they allow for additions and deletions. It is also a good idea to have separate manuals for policies and procedures as they convey two very different types of information. There are times, however, when a policy statement will need to refer the user to a specific procedure and vice versa. Before the manuals are put together, the overall organization must be given careful thought. Remember that well-organized manuals will be used more frequently because they will not frustrate the user. Many health care institutions use a numerical system for their manuals. For example, the 100 numbers in a policy manual would contain patient care policies; the 200 series, personnel policies; the 300 series, organizational or administrative policies; and so forth. Such a system allows for additions or deletions in the series without disrupting overall manual organization. In addition, policies and procedures should be dated to facilitate the review and revision processes.

Policies and procedures should be carefully written and edited at several levels to be certain that the content is accurate, clearly stated, and easily interpreted. In addition, you should choose words which are understood readily by all members of the audience and avoid the tendency to overwrite. Length is sometimes a deterrent to usage. Manuals that are unclear or difficult to understand will not be taken seriously and may promote organizational chaos due to multiple interpretations.

A final general consideration in the development of policies and procedures is that provision must be made for regular review and updating of manuals. This process should take place at least once a year and could easily be accomplished by committees established within a department. These committees might also be charged with drafting new policies and procedures as they become necessary. The committee might consist of two or three management personnel (supervisor, head nurse, etc.) and several staff nurses who want to become managers. The input of these staff nurses is invaluable as they are the persons most likely to be using the manuals.

WRITING POLICIES

The task of determining appropriate content for a policy manual is not easy. The tendency to write a policy for every possible issue that may arise is inadvisable because it may deflect attention from serious issues, and it may result in a manual that is too bulky to be readily used. In addition, this practice may stifle the development of decision-making skills of the nurse manager. How, then, is content determined?

First, consider that a policy provides guidelines to employees in recurrent situations. This authoritative source of readily available information helps to provide a locus of structure and control without the need for consulting the nurse manager. Policies may clarify areas of responsibility or provide a basis for delegation of decision making. Three general areas often addressed in nursing policy manuals include areas of responsibility related to specific patient care activities, protection of rights of patients and families, and personnel considerations. Other sources of policy include guidelines from accrediting agencies and policies addressing the implementation of institutional mission and goals.

Begin a policy with a subject heading. This will aid in the organization of the manual and the index. A brief statement of purpose following the subject heading will help the reader identify the reason for the policy. The actual text of the policy statement should follow these introductory sections. Content of the statement must be consistent with the stated purpose. (This seems obvious, but we have seen many policies in which content and purpose seem to bear no relationship to one another.) And, of course, the policy should be congruent with the institution's mission and goals and with other policies.

Avoid basing policies on personal biases or preferences. (A good example of this would be a restrictive dress code policy.) Also, guard against the tendency to develop policies around the "we've always done it that way" philosophy. Finally, when writing a policy, consider the feasibility of implementing it in your work setting. Don't expect the impossible or unreasonable.

When the need for a policy statement on a particular issue becomes apparent, the Director of Nursing should delegate the responsibility for drafting the policy to the Nursing Service Policy Committee. The next step is to review the policy. Some health care institutions have guidelines (or a policy statement) regarding the review and implementation of a new policy. In the absence of these guidelines, the policy should at minimum be reviewed by nurse managers of the areas directly affected by the policy, the Director of Nursing, and, *as appropriate,* institutional committees such as a medical-nursing joint practice committee, interdepartmental policy committee, or the hospital administrator. Remember that effective policy-making must include the support of all levels of management likely to be affected by the policy.

Examples of Policies

Let's consider some examples. Review each of the examples presented according to the guidelines described in this chapter. How would you change or improve these policies?

Nursing Service Policy #32

POLICY STATEMENT: The department of physical therapy will assume responsibility for transporting patients to and from their department for treatment as of 7/1/85.

Nursing Service Policy #118

8/3/75

SUBJECT: Scheduling of vacations

PURPOSE: To insure quality patient care

POLICY STATEMENT: All vacation requests must be submitted to Mrs. Alexander by April 1st of each year.

Nursing Service Policy #235

9/5/83
Review 7/84, 7/85

SUBJECT: Emergency treatment of cardiac arrhythmias in the intensive care units.

PURPOSE: To provide immediate treatment of cardiac arrhythmias in the absence of a physician.

POLICY STATEMENT: Registered nurses working in the intensive care areas and who have completed the emergency cardiac care course of the hospital or who hold certification from the American Association of Critical Care Nurses may institute emergency drug protocols (as described in procedures 343, 344, or 345) in the absence of a physician's order when a life-threatening arrhythmia is identified in a critical care patient.

Did you notice that the first example is not dated, nor does it contain a statement of purpose? In addition, did you wonder whether the physical therapy department was aware of this policy change and how they would be notified of a patient who required treatment?

The second has not been reviewed or revised in 10 years! The statement of purpose is very vague and uses the cliché "quality patient care." Did you wonder what would happen if Mrs. Alexander no longer worked for the institution? It's a good idea to identify positions rather than names in policy manuals. Finally, the subject is identified as scheduling of vacations, but the policy statement refers to vacation requests. You might wonder how and when those requests became scheduled vacation time.

The last example contains a date and indicates two reviews since its implementation. The subject and purpose are clearly identified and related to the policy statement. The policy statement clearly indicates who may do what, under what circumstances, and refers to specific procedures which may be consulted in order to properly carry out the policy.

Many health care institutions provide space for the review and approval of certain persons within the institution. For example, a policy might be signed by the Director of Nursing Service, a hospital administrator, and the chief of the medical staff. This is a point to be considered by each institution as it may aid in the enforcement of the policy. The following checklist provides you with a ready review of the important aspects of policy writing.

1. What is the source of the policy?
2. What is the purpose of the policy?
3. Does the policy conform to institutional mission and goals, preexisting policy, and guidelines of accrediting agencies?
4. Is the content of the policy clearly related to its purpose?
5. Is the title clear and easily indexed?

6. Is the content stated simply and clearly, or is there room for mis-interpretation?

7. Is the policy placed in the proper section of the manual?

8. What is the date of the policy? Should this policy be reviewed more frequently than every year?

9. Has the policy been reviewed and approved by the proper authorities?

10. Is there likely to be any difficulty with enforcement of the policy?

Distribution and Enforcement of Policies

When a new policy has been written and approved, it should be copied and distributed to all appropriate persons for placement in their manuals. The policy should be clearly identified by number so that it will be correctly placed in the manual. It's also a good idea to update the index yearly to reflect additions and deletions. A new policy should be accompanied by a cover memo announcing when it will become effective. This is a good way to call attention to the fact that a new policy has been enacted. In addition, it may be necessary to orient certain personnel as to their responsibilities related to a new policy.

It's important to stress again that for policies to be effective they must be enforced. Granted, there may be exceptions; however, these should be rare. If you find that exceptions are constantly being made to a certain policy, it may indicate a need for policy review and revision or a reminder of the need to enforce the policy.

WRITING PROCEDURES

A procedure differs from a policy in that it details *how* to do something, while a policy specifies who is responsible for doing something or what is to be done under certain circumstances. The differences between policies and procedures can be easily illustrated by using the situation in which a patient dies. Policies related to a patient death might include who should be notified, who is responsible for the death certificate, or under what circumstances an autopsy is required. Preparation of the body and care of personal belongings, on the other hand, would most likely be described in procedures.

Determining content of a procedure manual may be problematic due to the seemingly endless number of possible topics. There are several points to consider carefully. The first and most important is, *who is the audience?* Many health care institutions have procedure manuals that include such basic nursing skills as how to make a bed, take a temperature, or bathe a patient. As you might imagine, these manuals are bulky, may be disorganized, and are therefore seldom used. The important question here is, *why reinvent the wheel?* A good nursing skills text could be placed on each unit for use by nurse aides or student nurses. This text in most cases would do a better job of illustrating and describing basic patient care skills than a procedure manual. The result of this approach would be a procedure manual devoted to advanced nursing skills, little-used skills, and new skills. Procedures might also include institution-specific matters such as the name and location of supplies available for carrying out certain patient care activities, forms relating to these activities, or physician requests for certain supplies in special care areas.

A second consideration when preparing a manual is that not all procedures need to be available on all units. For example, orthopedic procedures detailing use of traction devices do not need to be in the coronary care unit's manual. If a patient is admitted to coronary care with an additional orthopedic problem, the best approach would be to consult an orthopedic nurse rather than try to set up a complicated traction device based on an unfamiliar procedure. Careful analysis of your procedure manual based on these suggestions will result in a manual that is useful and specific to a particular unit.

Procedure Format

Again, as with policies, the format of procedures should be consistent. Several things will need to be included as applicable. These are listed for you to serve as a quick reference and then each is described in more detail.

1. Title
2. Purpose
3. Brief description of the procedure, indications for use, referral to specific policies, and so on
4. Physical and psychological preparation of the patient

5. Expected outcomes, possible complications, patient monitoring, and precautions
6. Responsibilities of physicians or nurses during the procedure.
7. Obtaining supplies
8. Step-by-step description of the process with illustrations as appropriate
9. Recording the results of the procedure

TITLE

Think through the title of the procedure carefully so that it will clearly identify the nature of the procedure at a glance. In addition, consider how the title will appear in the index. Remember, the well-organized manual is more likely to be used.

PURPOSE

You can write the purpose of the procedure in a short statement. This will aid those unfamiliar with the procedure in understanding the reason for or objective of the procedure. For example, the purpose of the peritoneal dialysis procedure might read: *To remove waste products from the blood utilizing the peritoneal membrane as the site of exchange.*

DESCRIPTION OF THE PROCEDURE

At this point, describe the procedure briefly to aid the reader in understanding when to use the procedure. This is also a good place to refer to any applicable policies. Keep this section brief, since it is an orientation to the procedure and not a detailed description of the process.

PHYSICAL AND PSYCHOLOGICAL PREPARATION OF THE PATIENT

This section will aid the user in preparing the patient adequately for the procedure. This very important aspect is sometimes forgotten in the flurry of activity to get the "task" done.

EXPECTED OUTCOMES

The expected results of the procedure should be carefully described. This will help to determine the degree of success of the process and also will help to identify any complications. Special precautions, possible complications, and guidelines for patient monitoring will also need to be included.

RESPONSIBILITIES OF PERSONNEL DURING THE PROCEDURE

Certain procedures can be performed only by certain personnel. These should be carefully described so that there is no confusion related to roles and responsibilities. These descriptions will also need to be carefully checked to be certain that they do not conflict with policy statements addressing the same subject.

SUPPLIES

Necessary supplies should be listed in an organized fashion. Avoid the tendency to describe the location of supplies; these may not be applicable to all situations. Forms for requisitioning special supplies from other departments should be described here. For commonly performed procedures, many institutions have developed trays or packs that contain all of the necessary supplies.

STEP-BY-STEP DESCRIPTION OF THE PROCESS

This is the heart of a procedure. It should be well-organized and written clearly and simply. Information contained in previous sections should not be repeated here, as this should describe only what is needed to carry out the procedure correctly. Extraneous or nice-to-know information will only confuse the user and may result in incorrect performance. You may want to use illustrations to enhance the descriptions, but don't overdo it.

RECORDING

This will serve as a useful reminder to the user as to what should be recorded in relation to the procedure. Specifics as to the patient's condition, complications or difficulties encountered, and the psychological response of the patient are considered pertinent.

The following example of a peritoneal dialysis procedure illustrates the important aspects of procedure writing.

Title of the Institution
Department of Nursing

Procedure #365
TITLE: Acute Peritoneal Dialysis

PURPOSE: To clear the blood of waste and unwanted solutes using the peritoneal membrane as the site of exchange.

DESCRIPTION: Peritoneal dialysis is a process whereby waste products and unwanted solutes are cleared from the blood using the peritoneum as the membrane of exchange. Fluid (called dialysate) is introduced into the peritoneal cavity via a trocar or catheter. This fluid is allowed to remain in the cavity approximately 15–30 minutes where it collects solutes from the blood by simple diffusion across a membrane. The fluid is composed of many of the normal blood solutes such as Na^+, K^+, Cl^-, H_2O, etc. Dextrose is also used to influence the osmotic pressure of the dialysate and therefore help to restore fluid balance according to patient needs. When a patient is unable to clear solutes in the kidneys, the normal blood concentrations will rise. By exposing the blood (with high solute concentrations) to the dialysate with near normal solute concentrations, diffusion across the peritoneal membrane will in effect pull these excess solutes out of the blood. After a prescribed period of time (15–30 minutes) the dialysate is drained out of the cavity using gravity. The number of exchanges required during each session is determined by the physician and is based on the patient's condition.

Indications for use of peritoneal dialysis include renal failure (both acute and chronic), fluid and electrolyte imbalance, or drug overdoses. Peritoneal dialysis is slower and less effective than hemodialysis; however, it does not require the specialized equipment and personnel that are necessary with hemodialysis. A distinct advantage of peritoneal dialysis is that is does not cause fluid and electrolyte imbalances so readily and is therefore very effective in infants, children, and the aged.

PHYSICAL AND PSYCHOLOGICAL PREPARATION OF THE PATIENT:

1. Thoroughly explain the procedure and purpose to the patient and family.

2. Encourage questions and give the patient an opportunity to discuss his or her anxiety.

3. Assure the patient that pain medication will be available as needed, although the process is not usually painful but can be uncomfortable.

4. Describe the equipment, physical preparation, and nursing care that will take place during the procedure.

5. Empty the bladder by instructing the patient to void or by inserting a Foley catheter as ordered by a physician.

6. Shave and cleanse the abdomen.

7. Record baseline vital signs and weight.

EXPECTED OUTCOMES:

1. Vital signs and weight are stable.

2. Electrolytes and serum analysis are within normal limits. (Drug is cleared from blood.)

3. Fluid balance is restored.

4. The patient experiences no complications. Possible complications include perforated bowel or bladder, peritonitis, fluid and electrolyte imbalances, hypothermia, bleeding, hyperglycemia, and excessive pain.

RESPONSIBILITIES OF PERSONNEL:

Physicians: See policy #183.

1. Correct insertion of the catheter into the patient's abdomen.

2. Determine the amount and composition of dialysate.

3. Determine the number of exchanges.

4. Follow the patient's condition and response to the procedure.

Nursing Personnel

1. Prepare the patient both physically and psychologically. (RN)

2. Obtain supplies.

3. Carry out the exchanges. (RN)

4. Monitor the patient during the procedure. (RN)

5. Notify M.D. of unexpected changes in patient condition.

6. Assist the physician as necessary.

SUPPLIES: Obtain a peritoneal dialysis tray and a backup from the central service department using the standard requisition #00430. Order solution from pharmacy as specified by Doctor's order on standard pharmacy requisition #00435.

THE PROCEDURE:

1. Take baseline vital signs: BP, T, P, R.

2. Record patient's weight.

3. Empty patient's bladder by encouraging voiding or by Foley catheterization (per M.D. order).

4. Warm the solution to body temperature to prevent hypothermia.

5. Connect tubing to solution, remove air from tubing.

6. Clamp outflow tube.

7. Assist physician with surgical prep of the site and draping.

8. Prepare local anesthetic and an angiocath. *Note:* M.D. will insert approximately 1000cc of solution via angiocath to clear the bowel from the area before insertion of the dialysis catheter.

9. Prepare trocar and catheter for insertion into the abdomen.

10. Connect tubing to catheter.

11. Instill first 2000cc of dialysate. (Physician may order differing amounts depending on patient's situation.)

12. Secure catheter firmly to abdomen.

13. Allow solution to remain 15–30 minutes.

14. Drain slowly (over 20 minutes) by opening outflow valve.

15. Check dialysate for color and amount. (Inflow = Outflow)

16. Check and report diarrhea or bladder discomfort, which may indicate bowel or bladder perforation.

17. If necessary, medicate for pain or sedate as ordered by physician.

18. Take vital signs q15 minutes × 2, then q30 minutes × 2, and then q1 hour if stable.

19. Perform the number of exchanges as determined by the physician.

20. Report complications, poor fluid return, changes in vital signs, and other changes in patient condition promptly to the physician.

21. Assist the physician with trocar removal.

22. Apply topical antiseptic ointment to insertion site and apply a dry dressing. Change at least every day and more frequently if drainage occurs.

RECORD:

1. All vital signs and patient weight.
2. Patient's psychological and physical response to the procedure.
3. The number of exchanges, time of inflow and outflow, and amount of fluid utilized on Peritoneal Dialysis Flow Chart, #013.
4. Complications encountered.
5. Notification of physician.

You may find that you prefer a different format. One advantage to the format suggested here is that the actual steps in the performance of the procedure are separated from the background information, which provides for quick reference. The format you develop for your procedure manual should at the very minimum contain all of the information suggested here. Supplying the staff with this information will help to ensure confident and competent performance of the procedure.

9

Proposals

Do you have creative ideas that you would like to see implemented in your work setting? Do you avoid pursuing your ideas because you are aware of budgetary constraints? Have your ideas been repeatedly "shot down" or ignored by higher levels of administration? If the answer to any of these questions is yes, then you may need to consider proposal writing seriously.

A proposal is a means of outlining in detail a problem and your ideas for solving it. It is a formal way of presenting an idea to people with the power and resources to implement the idea. This chapter will examine proposal writing from two perspectives. The first is formal proposal writing techniques which you would use when submitting an idea to an outside agency such as the federal government or a foundation (Kellogg, for example) in order to gain funding. The second is the application of these same principles on a less formal basis for in-house proposals in order to gain financial support or other resources from the institution.

GENERAL GUIDELINES

One of the important things to remember when proposing a change that requires the commitment of scarce resources is that the competition is usually great. A well-thought-out and well-written proposal will not always gain approval, but you can be sure that a poorly organized and poorly written proposal may not even be read in its entirety. This is an extremely important time to *consider your audience.* Who is likely to be reading the proposal? How familiar are these persons with the nature of your proposal? Are you speaking the right language? Answers to these questions may or may not be found in guidelines published by the agency.

The second important rule is to follow the guidelines provided by the agency. For example, the Federal Register, January 23, 1976, contained detailed rules and regulations to be followed for the preparation of a training grant application for a Nurse Practitioner Training Program. In addition, the application packet obtained from the Department of Health, Education and Welfare contained detailed guidelines for preparation of the five-page printed application and the detailed program description. The table of contents of the formal proposal written according to these guidelines is provided here for your review.

Table of Contents

When guidelines exist, make sure you are addressing all aspects of the guidelines. Omissions of requested information shed doubt on the quality of the proposal. Avoid providing information not requested in the guidelines unless you feel strongly that there is an obvious gap in information that is requested. Provide additional information only when you believe it will convince the reviewers that you are the person/institution best equipped to implement a particular program.

A final general rule is to pay careful attention to information given about the evaluation criteria for proposal review. This information can often be used as a checklist during your final preparation to ensure that you have included all pertinent information. Consider how the following criteria on training grant application review from the DHEW 1976 program might help you prepare a proposal.

Grant applications are reviewed with regard to the following:

1. Evidence of conformity to prescribed program guidelines and regulations.

2. Evidence of sound planning before submission of the application.

3. Documented need for the project/program.

4. Project/program objectives are clearly identifiable, attainable, and will be measured.

5. The methodology for carrying out the project/program is feasible and clearly described.

6. The proposed budget items support the project/program plan and assure effective utilization of grant funds.

7. The capability of the applicant to carry out the proposed project.

8. The extent to which the project has joint program direction by qualified nurse and physician educators.

9. Plans for continuation, including financial support of the activity after termination of the grant.

When guidelines do not exist or are very general, your job as a writer becomes more difficult. At this point, it's important to use your expertise to convince the reader that you are the person with the talents to implement the program. A good rule of thumb is to never assume that the reader is an expert in the field. In other words your proposal should demonstrate adequately that you fully grasp the nature of the project and that you or your agency have the expertise to carry it out effectively. For example, the 1977 annual report of the W. K. Kellogg Foundation included this information for proposal writers:

Proposal Applications

To be considered for Foundation aid, an institution, agency, or organization should write a proposal letter or memorandum briefly describing the basic problem and the plan for its solution including project objectives, operational procedures, duration, and personnel and financial resources available and needed. The Foundation does not supply formal grant application forms.

Proposal letters are carefully evaluated by the Foundation. If the proposal is within the Foundation's guidelines and if Foundation resources permit consideration of the requested aid, conferences and staff investigations may follow and the organization may be asked to develop a more detailed proposal. Frequently, the Foundation seeks counsel from advisory committees and individual consultants in addition to utilizing the advice of its own professional program staff.

Proposal letters are given prompt consideration and should be addressed to: Secretary, W. K. Kellogg Foundation, 400 North Avenue, Battle Creek, Michigan 49016.

These guidelines are considerably less detailed than those used to prepare the Nurse Practitioner Training Grant proposal cited earlier.

Take a moment to review the proposal letter (which follows) written according to these guidelines. Note that the budget was included in the proposal body, whereas in the previous example the budget was outlined on the printed application form which accompanied the body of the proposal.

January 10, 1985

Secretary, W. K. Kellogg Foundation
400 North Avenue
Battle Creek, MI 49016

Dear Secretary:

The Greystone University Medical Center, a nongovernmental, not-for-profit institution, is seeking financial assistance for the development of a program to educate Adult Primary Health Care Nurse Practitioners and promote their utilization in the northeastern Illinois area. The commitment of the Medical Center to the delivery of complete and optimal health care services to all members of the community, the recognized need to improve availability and accessibility of health care through the expansion of primary health care services, and the belief that nurses prepared to function in expanded roles can enhance the team approach to the delivery of health care and provide quality preventive and maintenance services were the impetus for the generation of this program.

NEED

Factors operational in this community which support the need for Adult Primary Health Care Nurse Practitioners are the following:

1. The overall population in the area continues to increase (62% of the population is between the ages of 16 and 64).

2. There is an average family and general practice physician-to-population ratio of 1:4627 in this and two adjacent counties. The goal for this physician-to-population ratio in Illinois is 1:2222 as identified by the Illinois Academy of Family Practice Physicians, June, 1984.

3. In 1982, it was estimated (nationally) that of 200 million emergency room visits, only 20% were true emergencies. The 1984 statistics for utilization of Medical Center Emergency Room support this estimate: 80% of visits were nonemergent; 20% of visits were emergent. This widespread misuse of emergency facilities is due to poor use or inaccessibility of primary health care services.

4. Recently, 5000 steel workers lost their jobs in a major steel mill closing. The overall effects of this event are not yet apparent; the need for increased affordable health care services may be projected.

5. There is a trend toward expansion of primary health care services in the area as evidenced by the proposed expansion of existing facilities and proposed construction of new sites.

6. The closest facilities for the education of nurse practitioners are located 500 miles away. Officials of these programs indicate that applications far outnumber the available spaces in the programs.

7. A survey of health care institutions in 1984 estimated the need for 75 nurse practitioners in this area in five years.

PLAN

An educational program to prepare nurses to function as nurse practitioners would serve to meet the above identified needs. Recognizing that nurse practitioners for the most part represent a new approach to health care delivery in this community, there is a need to develop and implement the program in two overlapping phases:

Phase I—Planning: This phase will last approximately one year. It will include introduction of the faculty in the role of nurse practitioners in the Ambulatory Care Center, for their development and the development of the nurse practitioner role; and curriculum development and program planning.

Phase II—Implementation: This phase will last two years, during which time 20 nurse practitioners will be prepared.

OBJECTIVES

1. To improve the delivery of health care to the consumer by providing the personnel to promote a shift in emphasis from acute care to primary health care which will:

   a. Improve accessibility of health care services.

   b. Improve utilization of current health care services.

   c. Assist in meeting health care needs of an expanding population.

2. To provide nurse practitioners to assist in meeting the projected five year need in the area.

3. To provide an accessible educational opportunity for nurses who wish to further their education, expand their roles, and update their skills.

IMPLEMENTATION: (Procedures, Time Schedule, Resources)

Greystone University Medical Center provides an appropriate educational/clinical setting for the proposed program, not only because of its ideal location in the region, but also because of its many clinical facilities and services. In 1983, the Ambulatory Care Center provided services to an additional 12,000 patients over the previous year, and it is anticipated that this trend would continue if personnel to supply these increased services were available.

Professional resources to begin implementation of the program are presently available. Two nurses, one a master's candidate in Community Health and the other holding a master's degree in Clinical Nursing, will serve as program faculty and are prepared to begin serving in the Ambulatory Care Center. It is anticipated that these persons would be the stimulus for the expansion of Ambulatory Care Services through use of nurse practitioners and serve as primary developers of the curriculum for the proposed education program.

Other professional resources readily available are:

Position	Function in Proposed Program
Director of Nursing Service (RN)	Nursing Director of Program
Director of Medical Education (MD)	Medical Director of Program
Director of the Area Health Education Network (RN)	Advisory Committee
Associate Dean of Greystone University College of Medicine (MD)	Advisory Committee
Nursing Faculty of Greystone University (RN)	Advisory Committee
Physician in Ambulatory Care Center (MD)	Advisory Committee

The above persons would provide valuable input and direction from both the medical and nursing professions, a factor which would enhance the collaborative role and the team approach to the delivery of primary health care.

The following table outlines the projected budget for the proposed program:

Phase I		
Personnel: 2 faculty	$17,000 base each	
	5,219 fringe each	$44,438

Additional expenses	4,000 part time	4,000
(Travel, continuing		
education)	1,000 each faculty	2,000
Consultants		
(fees and travel)	1,500	1,500
Equipment, supplies		
audiovisual aides	5,000	5,000
Subtotal		56,938

Phase II

Personnel: 2 faculty	Reflects 7.5% inc.	47,770
1 clerical	8,200 base full time	
	2,517 fringe	10,717
Additional expenses		2,000
(Travel, continuing		
education)		
Consultants		500
Equipment, supplies		
audiovisual aides		2,500
Subtotal		63,487

Phase III

Personnel: 2 faculty	Reflects 7.5% inc.	51,342
1 clerical	Reflects 7.5% inc.	11,523
Additional expenses		2,000
Consultants		500
Equipment, supplies,		
audiovisual aides		2,000
Subtotal		67,365
TOTAL		$187,790

PROGRAM CONTINUATION

Continuation of the program at the end of the three-year period is anticipated. The program will be supported by a combination of institutional subsidy, student tuition and fees, and alternate sources of funding.

Please notify if further information is necessary. Thank you for your prompt attention to this proposal.

Sincerely,

Constance K. Allen

PROPOSAL FORMAT AND CONTENT

In general, proposals should contain the following components: a problem statement, a purpose, background information, objectives, method of implementation, evaluation method, description of personnel, resources and/or facilities, and budget. The extent to which you will use these will depend to a large degree on the specificity of the guidelines for the particular agency you are addressing. Each of the usual elements of proposal content will be described in the sections that follow. Examples of each element are excerpted from the Nurse Practitioner Training Grant Proposal referred to earlier.

The Problem Statement or Purpose of the Proposal

The problem/purpose statement should be a succinct statement of what the proposal is addressing. This is where the tone of the entire document is set. The reader is unlikely to continue if unable to identify what he or she will be reading about.

For example, "The purpose of this proposal is to seek financial support for the planning, development, and operation of an educational program for nurse practitioners." Note how this statement describes precisely what the proposal is about.

Background Information

The identification of need for the proposed project is described here. This is where you sell your idea to the reader by convincing him or her of the necessity of supporting your program. Provide specific documentation of need whenever possible.

The following summary of the background information presented in the example illustrates the kind of information that is useful to include to support the need for your project.

> The need for a Nurse Practitioner Program in the Greystone University area has been identified by demographic data, health data, present status of primary health care services, available educational opportunities for nurses, and results of a survey. The establishment of an Adult Primary Health Care

Nurse Practitioner Program would help to meet educational needs of nurses and most importantly would improve the delivery of health care to the consumer by promoting a shift in emphasis from acute care to primary health care in the following manner:

a. Improving accessibility of health care services

b. Improving utilization of present health care services

c. Assisting in meeting health care needs of an expanding population.

Financial assistance from the federal government is essential to establish the program. Continuation of the program after the project period is anticipated and will be accomplished by a combination of institutional subsidy, student tuition and fees, and the potential for university affiliation.

The survey referred to in the summary addressed current use and projected need for nurse practitioners in the region. In addition, a list of persons and their titles in the region who sent letters indicating their support of the proposed program also appeared in this section. Copies of the actual letters of support were placed in the appendices.

Objectives

Objectives are precise statements about what you will accomplish if the proposal is accepted/supported. As described in detail in Chapter 6, these should be written in measurable terms. This will facilitate the evaluation of the proposed project.

Project objectives for the proposed nurse practitioner program are established to correspond with the need for a nurse practitioner training program in this area. The proposed program will meet the following objectives:

1. To prepare registered nurses to function as nurse practitioners.

2. To promote the delivery of primary health care through the use of nurse practitioners.

3. To provide nurse practitioners to assist in meeting the five-year need projected by the questionnaire respondents.

4. To provide an educational opportunity for nurses who wish to further their education, expand their roles, and update their skills.

Method of Implementation

This component is important because it helps to convince the evaluators that you have the expertise to carry out the proposed project. Start with a statement of institutional clearance. Describe who has been contacted and what approvals have been granted. An actual letter of approval from appropriate members of the administration could be included in the appendices. This ensures that you have the support of your institution to pursue the project. Next, provide an overview of the project and a time plan. What will the project consist of? Who will be involved? What are the steps in implementation? When will each of these steps be accomplished? In our example, the general structure of the program and curriculum were described. This was followed by a detailed time plan which indicated the activities which would take place during the three-year project period. Included in this time plan were ongoing evaluation processes and planning for alternate funding sources for the continuation of the program. Finally, the method of implementation section included descriptions of the curriculum, objectives, student plans for recruitment and application procedures, plans for accreditation of the program, and faculty development activities.

The amount of detail necessary in the method section of a proposal will depend largely on the nature of the proposed activity and the guidelines provided by the funding agency. If the purpose of the proposal is to seek approval for first planning a certain program or activity and then implementation, the method section would address planning activities that would take place after proposal approval.

Evaluation Method

This is a critical element in any proposal, because it demonstrates that you are willing to judge the relative effectiveness of the activity that you are proposing and thus make a sound decision for the continuation of the activity. Sometimes, evaluation may take place before the actual proposal and implementation. This is usually the case when a proposal is addressing the purchase of equipment. A pilot evaluation of the proposed equipment would appropriately be included in the background information section of the proposal.

Evaluation methods used in the example include student performance in both theory and practice sessions, the extent to which curriculum objectives were met, collections of student and graduate data, and the extent to which project objectives were met.

The evaluation methods selected should flow logically from the objectives of the proposed activity. If you have difficulty describing appropriate methods of evaluation, perhaps you need to revise your objectives.

Personnel

Who will be involved in the implementation of the proposed activity? What is the anticipated administrative or supervisory structure? What are the qualifications of those involved? Are they currently employed or will personnel need to be recruited? If they are currently employed, how will project implementation differ from or mesh with current job responsibilities? Will additional support personnel need to be hired? Answers to these questions may also be a critical factor in the proposal review process. It's important to anticipate what the reviewers will be looking for in personnel and to describe in detail what specific qualifications of personnel will enhance proposal implementation. The degree of commitment and availability of highly qualified and experienced personnel may be a critical deciding factor in the review process.

In the example provided, the administrative structure was delineated and included an advisory committee and consultants in addition to the program directors and faculty. *Curricula vitae* of key personnel were included in the appendices. The body of the report provided a summary of qualifications of key personnel.

Again, the goal is to convince the reviewers that you fully understand the nature of the proposed activity and that you or your institution is prepared to assign qualified personnel in sufficient numbers to appropriately implement the activity.

Resources and Facilities

This section addresses current resources and facilities of the institution available to support the proposed activity. Depending on the nature of the proposal, this section may not be necessary. However, your institution may be able to provide office space, equipment, clerical support, and general overhead costs (such as electricity, telephone, and heat). These should be described. Including this information may help to convince reviewers of the extent of institutional support and commitment.

The sample proposal included library facilities, general overhead services, community resources, and a detailed description of the institutional facilities.

Budget

Your budget should present a clear and concise summary of how the requested money will be spent. It's wise to consult with your institution's financial officer to aid you in the preparation of the budget. Generally the budget information might include such areas as personnel salaries and fringe benefits, equipment (including maintenance and repair), supplies, staff travel and continuing education, facility renovations, and overhead costs. Once again, reviewers will be looking for proposals which clearly address reasonable anticipated expenses. If you believe that a certain item of your proposed budget might seem unusual, you should include a footnote explaining the important nature of this difference. Make sure that salary ranges are in line with the national or regional averages for that type of position. In addition, if the institution is prepared to absorb certain costs, be sure to include the category as a line item on the proposed budget with a footnote to this effect. This will ensure that the reviewers remember this commitment of the the institution described in the resources and facilities section. If the item is omitted, it may appear as though you forgot to consider it, and this could result in a negative review.

The example we considered earlier contains a proposed budget. Take a moment to reread this example. Here is an additional example of a breakdown of equipment costs from the training grant proposal. Note the use of footnotes to enhance the reviewers' understanding of budget items.

Equipment Costs (Note 1)			
	Number	Cost/Unit	Total
Office Equipment (Note 2)			
Desks	3	175.00	$ 525.00
Desk chairs	3	125.00	375.00

Equipment Costs (Note 1) (continued)			
	Number	Cost/Unit	Total
Office Equipment (Note 2)			
Side chairs	4	35.00	140.00
Telephones	3	40.00	120.00
File cabinets	3	150.00	450.00
Bookcases	2	65.00	130.00
Typewriter, IBM Electric	1	950.00	950.00
		Total Office Equipment:	$2690.00
Classroom equipment			
Blackboard	1	70.00	$ 70.00
Bulletin board	1	25.00	25.00
Chair desks	12	132.00 (4)	396.00
Conference table	1	115.00	115.00
Chairs	5	50.00	250.00
Lectern	1	200.00	200.00
		Total classroom equipment:	$1056.00
Audiovisual equipment (Note 3)			
Overhead projector	1	300.00	$ 300.00
Slide projector	1	250.00	250.00
Cassette tape recorders and players	3	40.00	120.00
Videotape player with TV screen	1	2500.00	2500.00
16mm movie projector	1	900.00	900.00
		Total audiovisual equipment:	$4070.00
Clinical laboratory equipment (Note 4)			
Diagnostic kits	2	150.00	$ 300.00
Triple-head stethoscope	2	35.00	70.00
Sphygmomanometers	2	50.00	100.00
Percussion hammers	2	5.00	10.00
Pocket lights	2	8.00	16.00
Tuning forks	2	10.00	20.00
Vaginal speculum	1	10.00	10.00
		Total laboratory equipment:	$ 526.00
		Total equipment costs:	$8342.00

NOTES ON EQUIPMENT COSTS

1. Physical space, alterations, and renovations are an "in-kind" service of the Medical Center.

2. Miscellaneous equipment such as file boxes, letter trays, etc., are an "in-kind" service of the Medical Center.

3. Audiovisual equipment is included to provide equipment that is always available to the Nurse Practitioner Program. Videotape player is requested without recorder as the Medical Center has a recording studio which is readily accessible, but the videotape players are heavily utilized and, therefore, may not be available.

4. Students will be required to purchase their own diagnostic equipment.

Remember when preparing a budget to review carefully the guidelines provided by the funding agency because they may contain specific instructions regarding allowable expenses. Additional information may also be found in the criteria for review of proposals.

Locating Potential Sources of Funding

Several sources provide information about the availability of federally assisted programs and private foundations. These include the *Catalog of Federal Domestic Assistance,* the *Federal Register*, the *Foundation Directory*, and *Grantsmanship News*. Also watch for reports of activities of federal and state legislatures which may indicate new sources of funding. Professional journals may include information about federal legislative activities related to the funding of projects in health care. University libraries are often another good source of information. In addition, many major universities have specific offices dedicated to finding funding for particular projects. On a local level the community library, local government officials, or Chamber of Commerce groups may have information regarding funding from local agencies or community interest groups.

IN-HOUSE PROPOSALS

Many nurse managers find themselves in the position of needing additional financial support, equipment, or personnel from their employing institution. Often, attempts at getting this support are unsuccessful. The nurse manager who uses the techniques described in this chapter may find that he or she will be more successful. It's quite easy to respond negatively to a verbal, informal request. However, it's quite another matter when requests are formalized, well-thought-out, and supported with specific information. Even if the proposal is not immediately approved, it certainly will have the effect of calling attention to the problem or situation addressed and may lead to further future consideration.

Not all proposals will be requests for money. Here is an example of a proposal to provide a specific service to families using existing personnel. It is appropriate to make such a request formally because the successful implementation of this program depends upon the support of the nursing and medical staff.

To: Associate Director for Nursing Service and Associate Director for Medical Services

From: Chaplain
Social Service
Clinical Nurse Specialist

Date: February 22, 1985

Re: Proposal to Implement a Support Program for Families of Critically Ill Patients

PROPOSAL STATEMENT: To establish a team which will provide support for families expected to be faced with participation in critical decision making about the welfare of a patient.

BACKGROUND INFORMATION AND RATIONALE: In the intensive care units families are sometimes faced with decisions regarding initiating and/or continuing therapy for critically ill patients. Since families generally have little experience and knowledge of medical-legal-moral problems and alternatives, and this process may cause guilt or family disagreement, the nursing staff often call for assistance from the chaplain, social service, or a clinical nurse specialist to support the family. The difficulty with current practice is that the family may not know the persons called to provide support and assistance, and therefore the effectiveness of this support is minimal.

The specific situations which provided the impetus for this proposal are:

A. Removal of life-support system when brain-death has occurred.

B. Decisions not to pursue extraordinary means of life-support (especially resuscitation).

C. Need for health care in an extended care facility.

Services presently available from other departments do not address themselves to these specific needs. For this reason this program is not a duplication of service, but an enhancement of services available.

The need for establishment of an early relationship with a family in crisis or impending crisis is justified because the development of trust will enhance the effectiveness of support during a crisis. This type of support may prevent or help to control guilt and anxiety reactions of family members.

ALTERNATIVES:

1. To continue present practice of calling for assistance when the crisis is identified. As described above, this is ineffective.

2. To have open participation by personnel of pastoral care, social service, and nursing departments. This is unacceptable because there is a need for an organized, consistent approach by persons experienced in dealing with these situations.

IMPLEMENTATION:

1. The team will consist of one specially designated member from pastoral care, nursing, and social services.

2. Upon approval of initial proposal, the team will be available to present the program to appropriate committees as directed by the administration.

3. The members of the team will introduce the program to departments who are likely to be involved in making referrals.

4. Referrals are expected to come from physicians, nurses, and social services and can be made directly to members of the team or by contacting their respective offices.

5. The daily contact with families will be individual or as a team as deemed appropriate. Additional contact will be made as requested.

6. The team will meet on a regular basis to review progress on each referral.

7. A detailed operating procedure will be developed to aid health care workers in making referrals.

8. Home follow-up by telephone is an anticipated part of the service.

9. This program is viewed as an extension of present roles and therefore requires no additional personnel or resources.

EVALUATION: Evaluation of the program will take place between three and six months after implementation. Evaluation will consist of:

1. Number of referrals.

2. Appropriateness of referrals.

3. Subjective analysis by team members.

4. Reaction of referring personnel to program.

Note that many of the elements described in the previous section are contained here. An additional section entitled *Alternatives* was included as a means of anticipating and refuting other options that might occur to reviewers. It may also be appropriate to include a section which lists specific persons within the institution who support the proposal. At the very least, any proposal should contain a formal proposal statement, background information, implementation method, and method of evaluation. If your institution has guidelines for proposal preparation and submission, obviously these should be adhered to.

It is also important to consider who is the appropriate person or persons to receive the proposal. If you do not receive a response in a reasonable length of time, it is appropriate to follow up with a memo requesting the opportunity to discuss the proposal in person. This may also be an important strategy when a proposal is rejected.

If your proposal is rejected, try to find out why it was unsuccessful. This information will be useful for future proposals, revision of the existing proposal, or determining a more appropriate time for resubmission of the proposal.

Several additional techniques may increase the chances of acceptance of an in-house proposal. The first is to outline the cost-benefit of the proposal to the administration; this is especially useful when you are requesting money or other resources. Second, describe any personal benefit to the administrator. If acceptance and implementation of your idea will provide a "feather in the cap" of the administrator, that's to your benefit. Show how it will happen. Finally, you may need to consider the impact of the proposed change on the institution, departments within the institution, and personnel involved. If you anticipate resistance, analyze the nature of the resistance and address how you will deal with it. These approaches further illustrate the importance of the proposal and your ability to plan and implement it effectively.

10

Samples
for Analysis

In the pages that follow, we offer some examples of writing we and our students have collected. All of them are real. Each selection is (or is part of) a document that was written and circulated in a health care institution. All of them have gone wrong in one way or another, sometimes many ways. Most are not reader-centered. They fail to take into account the needs, attitudes, and knowledge of their intended audience. Indeed, the one addressed to "all concerned" shows no sense of audience whatever. We wonder how such a memo would reach appropriate readers: How do you know whether you're concerned by a memo until *after* you have read it? Most of the documents seem poorly planned. At least one (the new policy on changing IV tubing) was apparently reviewed and approved by two separate committees before being sent out, yet it strikes us as largely incomprehensible. Perhaps the rest of that institution's policy (or procedure) manual is written more clearly. We hope so.

Some of these examples are unintentionally funny, some merely confusing, and one or two could actually be dangerous. Even experienced nurses would have some difficulty following the instructions they contain. And almost everyone, we think, would be aggravated by the mistakes in tone and style made by these writers. Because we don't want to embarrass anyone, we've deleted the names of the writers and their institutions.

All the selections are printed exactly as they were sent out and preserve the mechanical errors of the original. We've marked each example with small letters that lead you to our comments and questions below. We'd like to thank the many students who have offered us these (and other) samples. To protect the innocent, however, we won't name names.

[From a procedure for using a multi-lumen catheter]

4. If any lumen is unused or only used intermittently, it must be kept

A   patent by:

    a. Continuous drip of saline or heparin saline solution.

B   b. A heparin lock (will eliminate the need for KVO fluid, lines and
bags). (Flush solution is 100 units of heparin per ml. saline.)

       1) The heparin lock is reheparinized every eight hours.

       2) When lumen is used, the heparin lock is flushed with normal
saline (10cc) before administration of IV therapy and again immediately after administraiton of the IV therapy.

       3) Heparinize the lock to keep patent by injecting heparin solution
(100 units heparin/1ml normal saline).

C   NOTE: The "Dead-space" volumen of the lumens is as follows:

       Proximal Lumen (white hub)   0.35cc

       Middle Lumen   (blue hub)   0.35cc

       Distal Lumen   (brown hub)   0.50cc

A. The first line of step 4 seems to suggest that both a *and* b must be done to keep the lumen patent. To avoid confusion, the sentence probably should have been phrased *must be kept patent by either of the following procedures:*

B. Based on these instructions, what would an average float nurse do to keep the heparin lock patent?

C. Why is this information here? What purpose does it serve?

[A memo from a nursing administrator to staff nurses]

A   Should a patient have a series of nursing transfer summaries, please continue to record the summaries on the N₅ patient progress record <u>but</u> have
the summaries follow each other on the same N₅ patient progress record.
This will provide the nurse with a readily accessible synopsis of the patient

B   hospital and should more easily accomodate the capsulized synopsis necessary for the discharge summary. You may then record the discharge
summary on the same sheet of paper as the subsequent transfer summaries.
The transfer/discharge summaries can be located in the chart at the end
of the nursing section. Thank you for your cooperation in this matter.

A. What we think this writer means is: *Please record all transfer and
discharge summaries for each patient in sequence on the same form;
don't use a separate sheet for each summary.*

B. This language is so inflated that it obscures the meaning the writer
seeks to convey.

[A memo from a storeroom supervisor]

A   To: All Concerned
Subject: INVENTORY OF THE STOREROOM—PURCHASING

B   There will be NO purchase order numbers given out on Friday, June 29, 1984 as we will be taking our inventory of the Storeroom.

C   The only exception is an EMERGENCY all others must wait until Monday, July 2nd.

Your cooperation in this matter would be greatly appreciated.

D   Thank you and have a Happy Inventory to you too.

A. Who, precisely, should receive this memo?

B. What does this mean? Are only purchase order numbers affected by the closing of the storeroom?

C. Why would anyone need an emergency purchase order *number*?

D. What does this final sentence add to the meaning of the memo?

[From a procedure for preparing patients for a CT abdomen scan using an iodine-based dye]

A   IF THE PATIENT HAS A HISTORY OF IODINE SENSITIVITY, THE CT DE-
PARTMENT SHOULD BE NOTIFIED BEFORE ADMINISTERING THE ORAL
HYPAQUE MIXTURE.

B   3. One and half hours before the procedure, a mixture of 20ml of Oral
Hypaque mixed with 500ml of artificially sweetened Kool-Aid is given
orally.

A. Is the oral Hypaque administered after the CT staff is notified,
or does this really mean: *If the patient has a history of iodine sensitivity, call the CT department for instructions.*

B. This instruction could be interpreted in any of the following ways:

1. 20 ml Hypaque in 500 ml Kool-Aid given 1½ hours (90 minutes) before the procedure.

2. 20 ml Hypaque in 500 ml Kool-Aid divided and given in two
doses: one hour before and 30 minutes before the procedure.

3. Two doses of 20 ml Hypaque in 500 ml Kool-Aid each given
at one hour and at 30 minutes before the procedure.

[A memo announcing a revised policy on changing IV tubing]

A   SUBJECT: CHANGE IN IV TUBING CHANGE POLICY

A change in policy related to IV Tubing change was recommended by the Infection Control Committee and Approved by the Medical Executive Committee.

B   Effective April 5, 1983 the primary IV administration set will be changed every <u>odd calendar</u> day (1, 3, 5, 7, 9 etc. days of the month) with the addition of the first new bottle of IV solution ordered and administered after 12:00 Midnight. The only exception to this policy will be the IV nitroglycerin. In this case, the date the nitroglycerin is started should be

C   documented on the Kardex and the tubing only changed if the solution is running longer than forty-eight (48) hours.

D   The change in policy will certainly be more cost effective and the center for Disease Control has indicated that tubing only needs to be changed every forty-eight (48) hours.

E   To facilitate the process and reduce paper work which would be required to record dates and times on the Kardex, it was proposed that all tubing be changed on specific days of the month; therefore every odd calendar day was selected. Some tubing may be changed two consecutive days in a row, however it was felt that developing a routine to change all primary tubing on the same day might facilitate the process and reduce record keeping.

F   Red and blue tape will be used to denote a tubing change with a switch to the opposite color when the change is made.

> Example: Red Tape—1–5–9–etc.
>   Blue Tape—3–7–11–days of month

The responsibility for changing the administration set is the nurse assigned to the patient and the procedure must be documented in the nurses notes.

G   The revised policy will be forthcoming. Your cooperation in reducing hospital costs is appreciated.

A. More careful wording could have avoided the repeated "change" in the subject line.

B. This wording is very confusing.

C. Why is nitroglycerin treated differently?

D. Why are cost-effectiveness and the recommendation of the CDC in the same sentence?

E. Does this paragraph add any essential information that hasn't been covered elsewhere?

F. Assuming you figure out how to do routine IVs, what color would you put on nitroglycerin on the 5th of the month?

G. Should this be a procedure instead of a policy?

[A memo to nurses and physicians from a hospital laboratory]

A   RE: AVAILABILITY OF PROCAINAMIDE AND N-ACETYL-PROCAIN-
AMIDE

Procainimide and N-Acetyl-procainamide are performed in-house. The
B   test is routinely performed during the day time shift and results will be
available at 2:00 P.M. daily, 7 days a week. Venipuncture service is avail-
C   able throughout all shifts to provide the collection of peak and trough
D   levels.

A. Is this an accurate subject line?

B. Not until the second sentence does the memo indicate that it
concerns a newly available *test* for procainimide levels.

C. Does the last sentence make clear what it means? Peak and trough
levels of what?

D. Is this appropriate for a memo, or should it have been announced
as an addition to a procedure manual?

[A memo sent to physicians and nurses from a hospital laboratory]

RE: Semen Analysis (Sperm Tests)

A   As requested in our first issue of <u>LAB FOCUS</u>, microbiology requests that all semen analyses be scheduled with the section. Because of the lengthy, labor intensive procedure, specimens should be submitted on M–F 8:30
B   AM–Noon and 1–2:30 PM.

In addition, please comment if the specimen is for a complete sperm analysis or a post-vasectomy analysis. Complete semen analyses require the
C   normal lengthy procedure. In contrast, post-vasectomy checks require a quick procedure just to report the presence or absence of sperm.

In our continuing effort to control costs, provide faster results, and maintain quality patient care, your cooperation with our requests would be greatly appreciated.

A. Why was the initial information disseminated in LAB FOCUS (which we assume is a newsletter)?

B. Is the humor intentional or unintentional?

C. Since it's emphasized for a second time, we wonder just what the "normal lengthy procedure" involves.

Index